Quantum Body Sculpting

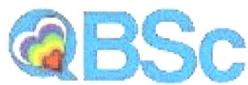

QBSc

From the inside out

A comprehensive program of

movements, procedures and meditations

for a complete body make-over

to captivate the joy of ageless living.

Trudy Baker QHP, QHI

Praise for Quantum Body Sculpting

"What if I could give my body a second chance at being healthy, having a perfect weight and all the energy I need to get on with my day? With QBSc I got all the tools I need to do just that and more.
A full weekend of exercises and meditations. I invite everyone to have a look at this pro-active health program."

Diane M. Brampton, Ontario

"It's fantastic, so full of energy charging, so much fun keeps you going and youthful...
It is fun and pro-youthing; keeping or reminding the body cells to remember their youth."

Miriam O. Laredo, Texas

Published by IEHealers Limited
All rights reserved.
Printed by CreateSpace
Available on Amazon and other online stores
Also available on Kindle

ISBN: 978-0-9916848-6-1

DEDICATION

To all women of all ages who like to look good and feel good.

We are offering you a way to use
your heart, your mind and your hands
to improve the way your body looks.

for the beauty of it

we use our hearts, minds, and hands to access
the Life Force Energy to sculpt our bodies

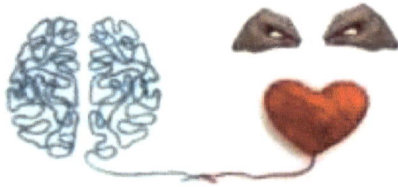

CONTENTS

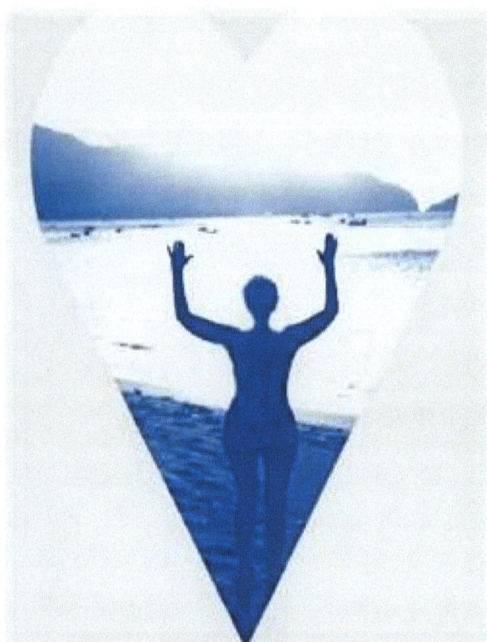

Quantum Body Sculpting

Why Body Sculpting?

Don't we all love a compliment about how we look, now and then? I do. It always makes me feel good when I do receive one. My entire body responds, smiling from the inside out. It was quite recently that I received an unforgettable compliment from my husband, one I will not likely forget.
We had been at an event where the people attending were of mixed ages. On the way home Everett said to me: "I know you were by far the oldest woman present at the party." He waited a bit before going on. A pregnant pause? I did not respond but waited for him to break the silence. He did, with the greatest of all smiles: "I also know and much appreciate that you were the best looking woman there. ☺ " I enjoy keeping myself in shape and having Everett compliment me on the way I look.

In the Quantum Body Sculpting program, I will share with you what I have done to stay in shape. It's been a lifetime practice which I have maintained through all my life's stages.

So, Why Body Sculpting? If you are in excellent shape now, the QBSc program will help you to maintain your good looks. If life's journey has caused you to lose your youthful figure and you would like to have it back, QBSc will help you. Using the techniques, doing the movements and exercises, listening to the meditations, and setting your intentions may well be a way to have compliments coming your way about how well you look, now and again, for as long as you live.

You will learn to tune into your inner self with the use of Meditations with Movement to resonate with positive vibrations and bring your body into balance with all energy systems around you. You will learn to allow all memories of your proportionate shape to resurface for you to look good today and into the future.

We show you how to release long-held non-beneficial thoughts and to rewrite any 'non-beneficial internal tapes' to maintain or re-create an anatomically correct and proportionately pleasing body shape for you. Our efforts are guided by intuitive, spiritual and holistic ideas from the heart. Whenever you are ready for the adventure, our course in body awareness and body sculpting is for you.

Be Beautiful.　　　　Be Well.　　　　Be You.

The Origin of Body Sculpting

The Quantum Face-Lift (QFL) program was a great success and several of our friends asked, "Why stop with the face? Why not give a lift to the entire body?" Miriam and I started brainstorming. We instantly knew we could do it. In the QFL program we are taking some of the age out of our faces. In Quantum Body Sculpting (QBSc) we are focusing on taking away some of the **signs of aging in our bodies.**

We knew that using similar techniques we used in the QFL program would work in the QBSc program as well.

To sculpt anything means to give shape to something.

A sculptor is an artist who creates statutes out of solid material. An artist needs to understand the media he/she is using.

For us, the medium is our own bodies. The tools are the love of our hearts, our intention, and the power of the Life Force Energy.

Quantum is a word taken from physics, quantum physics. I am not starting with giving a lecture on Quantum Physics. I want to mention that for me, the use of the word Quantum means that in the sculpting work we do, subtle changes will begin to happen at the most profound and deepest level of our existence.

Reading the book may well encourage you to plan to attend a workshop or a retreat and take the opportunity to be part of a complete Quantum Body Sculpting experience as well as share with and learn from a group of like-minded people. Enjoy a Participatory Weekend Workshop or choose to indulge in an All Inclusive 10-day Retreat in Costa Rica. Once learned, Quantum Body Sculpting will prove to be an excellent addition to anyone's fitness routine. For professionals working in spas, massage practices, anti-aging and wellness centers worldwide, QBSc is a powerful addition to your any professional repertoire.

Quantum Body Sculpting is an effective way to rejuvenate the body, to reverse the aging process, and to experience ageless living.

Who wouldn't like to have bragging rights about:
– firmed-up underarms
– smooth properly hydrated skin
– the total recession of varicose veins
– strong knees and ankles
– shapely calves, inner thighs, and buttocks
– firm, toned breasts
– a flat belly
– a trim waist-line
– a positive self-image

12

The Quantum Body Sculpting and the Quantum Face-Lift programs are easy to learn as stand-alone programs. There are no prerequisites other than a willingness to be open to new ideas and a new approach to caring for oneself. Both QFL and QBSc are participatory programs where one needs to take responsibility for doing the work oneself to have a level of success. What you will get out of doing the practice is directly proportionate to the effort you are putting into it. Neither QFL nor QBSc are the one and end-all of being healthy and well, to being beautiful and having an anatomically correct and proportionately pleasing body shape. Neither reading this book nor taking the workshops nor attending a retreat are guarantees to give you life-long beauty. Being healthy and well takes a total commitment to life-long self-care on all levels of one's being. Combined with exercise, nutrition, and meditation the QBSc and QFL programs will give you self-confidence about how you look and who you are now and into the future.

Learning to use Quantum Body Sculpting has the potential for an upgrade in your life. As a Wellness Coach, incorporating Quantum Body Sculpting into your practise, will exceed any expectations you ever dreamed possible.

Personally, I am convinced that my body wants to be healthy and well, and given half a chance it wants to remain so for all of my life. It's up to me to give myself that opportunity. My body responds to how I treat it, to the food I eat, to the self-talk I speak, as well as to the emotions I hold and emit.

So many of us go around saying or thinking: "Well, I'm getting older you know. What can I expect?" So many of us readily accept the limiting beliefs that are prevalent in our culture. 'With age, we can expect deterioration.' But is that necessarily true? What if we improve with age? Like good wine? I like to think that as I age, I get better. I am gaining insight to augment my eyesight. I am accumulating understanding to amplify my hearing. I am growing in wisdom to deepen the love in my heart.

I ask you to be open-minded to a new approach to well being. I encourage you to take responsibility for how you look and who you are in all the areas of your life. I invite you to be an artist and sculpt your own body.

Some Results You Can Expect

I taught the QBSc movements and exercises as part of an earlier workshop named Core and More several years ago. During the six months it took to put the program together, my husband and I practiced the QBSc movements and exercises. We began to feel more fit and continued the practice for months on end. My older sister had told me on occasion that I was beginning to stoop when walking, but I paid little attention to her well-intended mothering. It was not until I started looking at pictures of myself that I noticed aging showing in my posture. To my surprise, when I continued looking at pictures taken a year later, my posture had visibly improved. I give credit to the months of QBSc exercises and movements repeated and repeated until I knew they were effective and I was comfortable to teach them to anyone.

Changes took place in my posture after a year of Body Sculpting work.

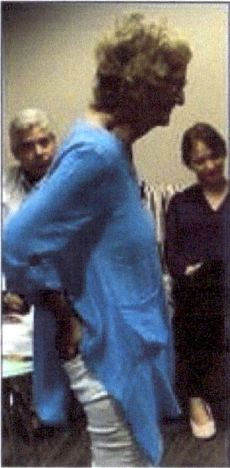

at age 77

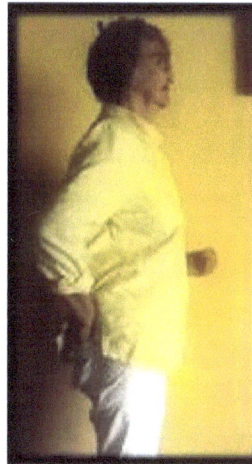

at age 79

Note: These pictures were NOT done by Sandoval El Bello Arte photography.

Comments written by a participant in one of the early workshops where I taught the Body Sculpting techniques.

I am basically skeptical in my approach to alternative healing. I tend to reserve judgment on the many various explanations provided by practitioners. For me, my personal experience is the proof in the pudding. This is what happened to me. I began with doing some of the Body Sculpting exercises described as 'Elongations with a Towel'. Initially, the imprint of my shoulder blades on the yoga mat was less than 2 inches; after several practice sessions, I could clearly identify the imprint as that of a human shoulder blade. Mine.

The healing definitely 'spilled over' in other areas of my life. I experienced radical healing from early childhood experiences. I experienced a positive improvement in some difficult inter-personal relations, confirmed to me by another person.

When I was home again after the workshop some friends said to me, "That weekend away was good for you. You look 10 years younger."

A New Way of Wellbeing

Why do **You** Want to do Body Sculpting?

Please take a moment to reflect on the questions below and jot down your thoughts about your body shape.

Is your body shape the way you want it to be?

Where on a scale of 1-10, where one is awful, and ten is awesome, would you put yourself?

Where on the scale would you like to be?

What would you be willing to do to achieve that level for yourself? Write down your answers and save them for now so you can later come back to them to measure your progress.

For you to get where you want to be the Quantum Body Sculpting program may well be the right answer.

Caring for our bodies

When doing the Quantum Body Sculpting, we are doing energy work with the use of some techniques chosen from several energy healing modalities. One does not need to be proficient in or committed to energy work. Just be open to trying some of the techniques which in some way often are very much like everyday activities we all do and use intuitively.

Your access to and use of the Life Force Energy may well be considered your most important resource when doing body sculpting work. While reading the book and doing the techniques, you will learn how to more readily access and make use of the Life Force Energy. You will learn how to use your heart to access it, your mind to direct it, and your hands to apply it. You will learn to pay more attention to many things you now do without thinking. You will learn how to focus and put your heart, mind and body to work for your highest good.

What follows is an introduction to how you can apply the benefits of the Life Force Energy. It is the enormous source of power available to all people, which we all use even without ever having heard of it or given it any thought. If you are familiar with doing energy work such as Reiki, Quantum Touch, Pranic Healing or similar modalities you may fast forward to 'How Body Sculpting Happens.'

"Self-approval and self-acceptance in the now are the main keys to positive changes in every area of our lives."

Louise Hay

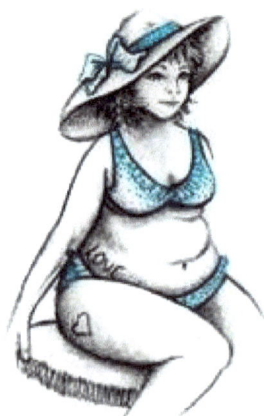

I believe my body is beautiful, and my body responds to that belief

Self Knowledge

A few questions

There are some questions to ask yourself before continuing to read and before starting on the QBSc program. The reason for these questions is the same as for any artist who works with any medium, whether it is wood or clay or metal, for sculpting. The artist needs to know the properties and the limitations of the medium before starting to work with it. If you are going to sculpt your body, you need to know the features and weaknesses of your body. What can you reasonably expect? The answers to the questions you give are for yourself only. Be brutally honest.

Please rate your answers to the following questions on a scale of 1 – 10, one being low, ten being the best possible.

- How well do you know yourself?
- How well do you like yourself?
- How well do you accept yourself?
- How well do you respect yourself?
- How well do you love yourself?

Body Awareness

Here are some more exploratory questions. For the best results take some time to write out the answers for yourselves. Keep your answers. They will be helpful after doing the QBSc work for a few weeks. You may be surprised at how your answers may change. Without keeping a record, you won't know how much you have changed.

How aware are you of your body?

If you are familiar with human anatomy, any question like: 'Do you know the location of your kidneys' may be silly. If, however, you do not know the location of your body organs I recommend you do some reading and become familiar with your body. Then answer the following questions. Enter a meditative space to find your answers. Can you feel your finger without looking at it? Can you feel your nose, your toes, your ears without touching them? Can you feel your heart without touching your chest or pulse? Can you sense your kidneys, your liver, your muscles when they are not aching? Take a journey through your body and become familiar with it on a new level. Keep a record of the experience and your feelings.

Have you learned to live with any tensions or limitations?

Depending on your current age, I invite you to think back ten years, twenty years or more. How did your body feel then? Were there any tensions? Limitations? What activities did you do then which you do not do now? Were they fun to do? Why are you not doing them anymore? Think of running, jumping rope, climbing a tree, participating in sports, working out. What made you stop doing those activities? Why? Would you like to be able to do those activities again? How would you feel doing them? Record your answers and impressions.

Are you wondering how to access your tensions and limitations and how to release them?

For many of us, when our bodies ache we either take a rest or push ourselves on in spite of the ache. Some of us take an aspirin or similar pain pill and hope for the aches and pains to go away. If they persist, many of us will see a doctor and accept medications, perhaps even go on maintenance medications to dull the pain and learn to live with it. Isn't that what we have learned to expect? Isn't that what aging is all about? I beg to differ. What if it isn't? Have you ever wondered if there is an alternative to living with 'the limitations of aging'?

Are you willing to learn to change yourself?

For those of you who are open to try a new approach to aging, read on.

Are you willing to learn to sculpt and reshape your body?

The QBSc exercises, movements, elongations, and meditations will give you the opportunity to carve out a new way to be you.

Are you ready for new levels of freedom?

The Quantum Body Sculpting course addresses the removal of many irritating details about how our bodies have begun to look, by using a holistic and energetic methodology. You will learn to tune into your inner self with the use of Meditations with Movement so as to bring your body into balance with all energy systems around you. You will learn to allow all memories of proportionate shape to resonate within yourself. We show you how to release long-held non-beneficial thoughts and to rewrite any non-beneficial internal tapes to help re-create an anatomically correct and proportionately pleasing body shape.

Get a second opinion

For some people, it may be beneficial to get a second opinion concerning some of the above questions you answered about self-knowledge. I don't mean for you to go ask a friend or relative or your health coach to give you an opinion about the accuracy of your answers. I invite you to get a second opinion from your own subconscious mind. If you recorded your immediate gut-felt or heart-felt answer the advice from your subconscious mind will likely validate your responses. If you stopped and considered, thought about the question before jotting down your response, it was your conscious mind answering, provided by your intellect. It was the answer you wanted to hear. Muscle testing is a method to get in touch with your subconscious mind, which drives your motivations based on values and beliefs learned at an early age. If your subconscious mind disagrees with your conscious mind, any program of self-improvement is likely to be sabotaged by limiting beliefs held at a subconscious level.

If you are familiar with muscle testing, I invite you to check your answers to these questions:

- How well do you
  o like?
  o accept?
  o respect?
  o love yourself?

If your answer to the first question was 9 for example, rephrase the subject as a positive statement. "On the scale of 1 to 10, where 10 is 100%, the answer 9 to the question 'How well do I like myself?' is correct." Do the same for the other questions. If you get a 'yes,' "Congratulations!" If you get a 'No,' I invite you to learn to balance and bring agreement between your conscious and subconscious mind. The technique of balancing is taught in a modality known as Psych-K. Freeing yourself from limiting beliefs about your self-image will significantly improve your success in any self-improvement program you are doing now.

See Appendix A for a brief explanation about Muscle Testing.

See Appendix B for a short introduction to Belief Busting, a derivative of Psych-K.

Tools and Techniques

The tools we use in the QBSc program are our hearts, our minds, and our hands with which we access the Life Force Energy. The techniques we use to connect with the Life Force Energy are Controlled Breathing, Meditation, and Intention. Once we connect, we use our hearts, minds, and hands to access the Life Force Energy to sculpt our bodies.

The Life Force Energy

The Life Force Energy may well be considered our most important resource which can be tapped into while doing the body sculpting.

Many other words are used to describe the Life Force Energy such as:

Chi - Chinese
Ki - Japanese
Prana - Hindu
Healing Power of Nature – Hippocrates
Light or Holy Spirit – Christians
Mana - Hunas, and Polynesians
Bioplasmic Energy – Russians
Orgon - Dr. Wilhelm Reich
Universal Gur – Alchemists
Universal Fluid – Anton Mesmer
Animal Magnetism – Anton Mesmer
Ka – Egyptians
Pneuma – Greeks
Universal Life Power – Baron Ferson
Psychotronic Energy – R. Pavlita (Czech)
Kirlian Energy
Motor force – Dr. John Keely
Tellurium – Prof. G. Kieser
Biochimica Energy – Dr. O. Brunler
X-Power – L.E. Eemann
Fifth Power
Pyramid Energy
Innate Intelligence – D. D. Palmer
Bioplasm
Ethers
Morphogenetic Fields - Rupert Sheldrake
Astral Light
Auric Energy
Life Force Energy
Love

How energy work works

Energy healing was a part of my childhood experience. It came to me as natural as walking or talking. My mother and my aunt, as well as some others in the family to a greater or lesser extent, 'helped people' to get well. I watched, and I learned. I 'helped' a pet dog, who was hurting, get well again. One time I 'helped' my sister to clear a rather nasty eye infection by placing my hand on it and then, followed with a sweeping motion of my hands, as if I were expelling the inflammation. Her eye infection disappeared. Nevertheless, I considered myself an ordinary kid. Today I consider myself an ordinary person. I believe if I can do it, so can others. My approach to energy work is intermodal. Although I am now trained in many different modalities, I do not favor any one over another. I have experienced the ease and seamlessness with which several healing modalities integrate with each other to promote self-healing.

A thorough understanding of how energy works is not required to do Quantum Body Sculpting. Some basics will help you to appreciate what is happening when you are doing the exercises, movements, elongations, and meditations. I will provide you with a brief overview of some techniques and background information. It will help you to follow the practices and to learn to do them for yourself and even with others.

How to quiet the mind and relax the body

There are various ways to quiet the mind, which in turn will ease the body. As a result, subtle changes will occur on a cellular level.

1. Meditation techniques with intention are easy to learn. Start with finding a quiet space: no radio, TV, cell phone, etc. Family, friends, children or even pets may present a challenge. Sit in a comfortable position. A lotus position is not required, especially for people who do not have the physical ability to sit that way comfortably for an extended period of time. Begin to breathe a little more slowly than normal and you will find your quiet place inside. Focus on your heart space and imagine your breath is going in and out through your heart. Pay attention to the rhythm of your breathing and follow the up and down movement the breathing creates on your abdomen. (Abdominal breathing is a sort of prerequisite.☺ cf. my book 'Come Breathe With Us') Pay attention to feeling the breath going in and out across your upper lip. If any distracting thoughts come in, quickly acknowledge them, and immediately let them go. Say to yourself: "OK, I'm thinking about that now. It can wait till later." Focus your attention on your breathing again. Once you begin to feel more relaxed, find your place of highest focus. Internally say to yourself, "It is my intention to be in touch with the Life Force Energy." Stay with that thought for two minutes. Pay attention to how your body feels. You

may feel a warming sensation all over. You may feel a slight tickling sensation. You may, and very likely will begin to have a sense of connectedness with all that is. You may not feel anything at all. With some practice, you will learn to go through these introductory steps in less than a minute.

2. Some people may like to try what is called the 'sweep and breathe' method in Quantum Touch. Here is my version of it. Stand with your feet about shoulder-width apart and your knees slightly bent and relaxed. Have someone gently caress your skin with a feather, or imagine someone is doing it, starting at the feet and slowly moving upward to the top of your head. From there, move down across the shoulders, along your arms, and out your fingertips. Coordinate your breathing and the caressing motion. Breathe in when the feather goes up. Breathe out when it is going down. With some practice, you can do it all in your imagination, without imagining a person is doing the caressing or even without the imaginary feather. Just focus on creating an energetic warmth or prickling feeling all over your body. Just breathing slowly will do it. Enjoy the feeling. The feeling is your awareness of the Life Force Energy. Alternatively, pretend two feathers are floating around you to do the caressing as above.
Quantum Touch Level 2 works with heart energy. It's powerful.
Start with a few "body sweeps" as explained above, caressing the body with the feathers.
Then put all your awareness into your heart; feel the love. Do gentle imaginary feathery 'energy sweeps' through the heart: from the bottom of the heart to the top, from the

31

back of the heart to the front, from the front to the back, and sideways through the heart. Feel the energy flowing through your heart into all directions, expanding your heart space. Allow love and compassion to fill your heart space, more and more. Send the love to someone who needs healing.

For the Quantum Body Sculpting work, emit those vibrations of love to the parts of your body that you want to sculpt.

3. Personally, I like using my variation of a Shamanic Earth - Star Meditation to activate an intense awareness of the Life Force Energy. To begin, stand relaxed. Raise your arms with palms facing upward. Focus your thoughts on a favorite star, on the heavens or the Divine. Invite the energies of the sky to enter into your being, through the palms of your hands, through the crown of your head and every pore of your skin. Allow the sensations to flow through your body. Now bring your arms down with palms facing towards the earth. Focus your thoughts down into the center of the earth and invite the energy of the earth to enter into your being, through the palms of your hands, through the soles of your feet and every pore of your skin. Invite the energies of the skies and the energies of the earth to blend into your heart space and amplify them with the love of your heart. Pay attention to how your body feels.

You may do any of the above techniques with your eyes closed or open. To end the session simply draw your attention back to your surroundings and take in the natural sights and sounds around you. It will bring you back to the here and now. Neither one or the other of the methods is necessarily better or more easily accessible than the other. I invite you to try all three, play around with them, and you will know what works best for you.

Experiment. Wonder. Enjoy.

Each time before doing a Quantum Body Sculpting session tune into the Life Force Energy field using one of the methods above, or your own preferred way.

All three methods are available as guided meditations on my website: www.IEHealers.com.

How Body Sculpting Happens

Body Sculpting, in the root sense, means we are re-sculpting parts of our bodies to improve the whole. Sculpting our body means to shape, or re-shape our body to a form it was intended to be: the authentic and holistic shape intended for our highest good. So many of us have inadvertently and unintentionally neglected our bodies. We've been too busy, committed to a workplace where we sit or stand all day, and glued to computers, phones, and TV sets even after working hours. We've not taken the time to provide our bodies with movement and exercise. We've tried to save time by eating fast-food, denying our bodies the natural nutrients required to be healthy and well. We are surrounded by toxic environments and take it all in stride. Even those of us who are healthy and well may have adopted the belief system of a culture that assumes our bodies will degenerate with age. We've accepted the mindset promoted by a society that we will need a healthcare system to take care of us. We've run to a doctor to give us medications when our body gives us pain. To me, pain is an alert telling me I have to do something about an issue that needs to change. So many of us have given up our right and responsibility to take personal care of our health and wellbeing.

In a way, Quantum Body Sculpting is a healing process, a self-healing process. I see it as an opportunity to take responsibility for one's body, how it functions and how it looks. All body sculpting is self-sculpting. The work is self-participatory and requires active personal involvement. You become the sculptor of your own body. The Meditations with Movement have the intent to sculpt and heal your body. We are aiming to bring our body into balance with all energy systems around us. We are activating all memories of proportionate shape to resonate within ourselves. By using Yin energy, we bring in quietness. We are inviting healing to happen by being receptive to the Life Force Energy to bring about subtle changes. The movements, elongations, and exercises promote maximum energy flow. All the movements, elongations and exercises are Meditations with Movement with the intent to sculpt and heal our body. The guided meditations release long-held nonbeneficial thoughts and erase any nonbeneficial internal tapes. We are now ready to take back our power to care for ourselves and set our intentions to take responsibility for our wellbeing.

Our next focus is on the glandular system. We set our intention for the glandular system to work at optimal capacity for our highest good, in support of the exercises and the energy work we do to sculpt our bodies.

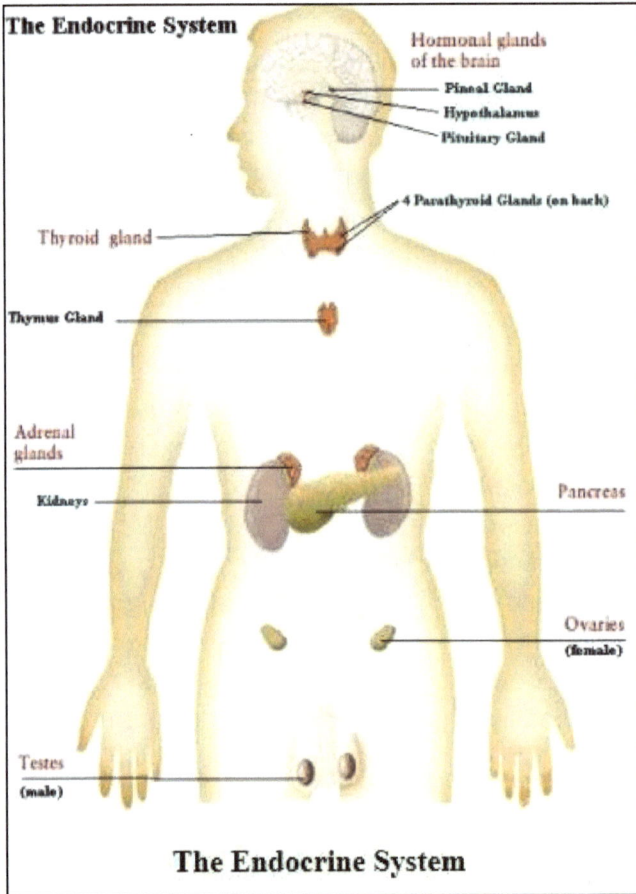

The Endocrine System

Hormonal glands of the brain

Pineal Gland
Hypothalamus
Pituitary Gland

4 Parathyroid Glands (on back)

Thyroid gland

Thymus Gland

Adrenal glands

Kidneys

Pancreas

Ovaries (female)

Testes (male)

The Endocrine System

By learning the position of glands in the body, you will know better where to focus your intention and, in some cases, where to place your hands.

The Glandular System

If you are well versed in human anatomy, you may wish to skip the following section and continue with reading 'The Benefits of Quantum Body Sculpting.'

The Glandular System, also known as the Hormonal System, consists of two parts: the Endocrine System, and the Exocrine System. Together they control and regulate just about every part of your body in very specific ways. They are responsible for your moods, disease resistance, and metabolism via the secretion of hormones. The endocrine system influences almost every cell and organ of the body. Some of the major glands of the endocrine system are:

- Pituitary gland
- Thymus Gland
- Hypothalamus
- Pineal Gland
- Thyroid
- Parathyroids

37

- Adrenal Glands
- Reproductive Glands (including ovaries and testes)

Why do we focus on the Glandular System when doing a Quantum Body Sculpting Session?

What does the Glandular System have to do with body shape issues?

A quote from Stacy on the www.refinebynature.com website pretty well sums up the answer to the above questions. "Leaders within the medical community, like Eric Berg, DC are finally clarifying body shape issues and their links to hormone imbalances in ways that the average person can understand. If you've ever had a hard time losing weight, keeping the weight off, have stubborn fat areas, gaining weight, or food cravings, I can guarantee that hormones are to blame. If you don't believe me, then think about the person you know who can eat anything he wants and can still stay skinny. How? Yes, it's his high metabolism, but hormones control metabolism, six fat burning hormones and three fat making hormones to be exact."

We engage the Life Force Energy to boost and in some cases reactivate the functionality of the hormonal system. When we "run energy" the energy follows our thoughts. Therefore, while doing Quantum Body Sculpting, think about your or your client's Endocrine System working at optimal capacity.

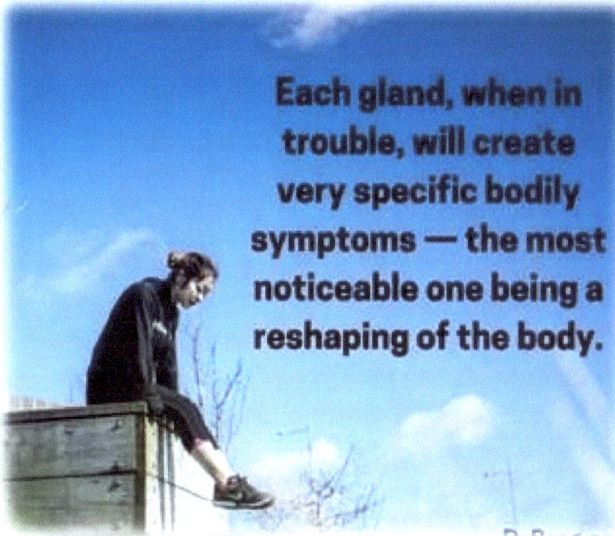

Each gland, when in trouble, will create very specific bodily symptoms — the most noticeable one being a reshaping of the body.

"Eric Berg is a health educator specializing in weight loss through nutritional and natural methods. His private practice is located in Alexandria, Virginia, with regular patients from the Washington DC and Maryland areas. His clients include senior officials in U.S. Government and the Justice Department, Ambassadors, medical doctors, high-level executives of some prominent corporations, scientist, engineers, professors, and other clients from all walks of life."

Although it is not necessary to know how all the glands work and what influence they have on your body shape, some familiarity with a few of the glands may be helpful.

The pituitary and the thyroid glands work together to regulate metabolism. The pituitary gland produces the Human Growth Hormone. It signals the thyroid to produce hormones which stimulate the growth of bone and other body tissues and plays a role in the body's handling of nutrients and minerals. If you have weight issues that cannot be corrected by an improved diet, or just by eating less if appropriate, focus your attention and set your intention on boosting the optimal functioning of the thyroid gland and proper communication between the pituitary and thyroid glands. cf: http://kidshealth.org/en/teens/endocrine.html

The pancreas is responsible for regulating blood sugar levels. It secretes insulin which helps glucose move from the blood into the cells where it is used for energy. Most people are aware that too much sugar and improper use of sugar in the body leads to weight issues. An intention for the pancreas to function at optimum capacity helps you to benefit the most from the body sculpting exercises.

The adrenals secrete about 50 different hormones including adrenaline and cortisone. The hormones from the adrenal glands control energy output and help us deal with stress. The adrenal glands are related to the stress we experience in our body. If a person experiences chronic, sustained stress, the adrenal glands begin to malfunction. The result is the accumulation of unwanted belly fat that the body mistakenly thinks is necessary to protect vital organs.

40

When breathing a bit more slowly than normal, repeating the positive affirmations like mantras and listening to the binaural background music on the meditations you experience a form of sound healing that strongly activates the pineal, pituitary and hypothalamus glands. Together, those glands regulate your physiology such as your metabolism, tissue function, growth and development, and ease of movement.

A QBSc practitioner received a note from a client to whom she had given a QBSc session.

It all started as small talk, but the truth is that QUANTUM BODY SCULPTING is simply "wonderful." I would doubt it if I did not see the tape measure myself. The therapy lasted no more than 20 minutes, and it reduced my waist by almost 3 centimeters. I sat there, with my mouth open. I could not believe it. It is a super therapy that not only helps you as a reductive therapy, but it also relaxes you, calms your anxiety and keeps you in a good mood. It is simply the best. Do not miss the opportunity.

J.A.G.

The practitioner's observation:

"I saw it with my own eyes. I measured it myself!!! I went, "Wait. What." And I re-measured it quite a few times just to be amazed over and over again. What a remarkable experience."

M.E.O

The Benefits of Quantum Body Sculpting

The benefits of a Quantum Body Sculpting session (QBSc) are manifold. People have experienced positive outcomes almost instantly. However, more commonly benefits become evident gradually over continued weeks of practice. Of course, it's not the same for everyone. Much depends on one's expectations and focus as well as on the commitment to continue with the program. It is never a one-time fix. It requires a commitment to self-care on a whole new level. It's comparable to any fitness program. We all know that one trip to the gym is not going to remove those unwanted inches from our waist-line, nor tone our legs and firm up our saggy underarms. Or think of a nutrition plan you've been advised to follow to improve your life. Reading a cookbook with many nourishing recipes is not going to do the trick. The Quantum Body Sculpting exercises and techniques work best with repeated practice. Do body sculpting in conjunction with a commitment to a healthy diet, and you have a winning

43

combination. Doing the program is an enjoyable experience. Try it; I guarantee no sweat, no sore muscles, and no outlay of a lot of money. Invest twenty minutes a day in yourself. The returns are phenomenal.

The techniques we use are non-invasive, and the results are soft and subtle. The slow breathing techniques will bring almost immediate relief of tensions and stress. They will help release long-standing rigidity in many parts of the body. Back pain, sinus issues, and headaches are likely to diminish notably. The meditative pace of the movements creates awareness of blockages, and with your intention, you will be able to release them. You will become aware of the limitations in your body that have crept in over the years. Your mind will open up to new possibilities. As well, the work on any particular areas of concern, such as unwanted belly fat and other fatty deposits will reduce the size of love handles or flabby flanks and reduce cellulite. Your muscles will firm up noticeably.

Guidelines

Wear loose and comfortable clothing when doing Quantum Body Sculpting. Take off all belts and other restricting items. Wearing simple track pants and a sweat-shirt or T-shirt may be most appropriate. Empty your pockets of wallets, coins or other bulky items. All movements and exercises are done barefoot on a yoga mat or a carpeted floor. Weather permitting, some may be done outdoors on a grassy lawn for extra grounding. The movements are very slow and non-competitive. Always move on the out-breath only. During exhalation, tensed muscles relax, and you can learn new routines without the risk of harmful stretching. When listening to the meditations sit in a comfortable and relaxed position in a location where you will not be interrupted. A lotus position is not required, especially not for those who are not comfortable sitting in such a way for any length of time. Working on areas of concern and body systems can be done with the eyes open or closed. Use a slight or near touch, without any pressure. The more relaxed the hands are, the better it will work.

No particular order for doing the program is preferable over another. It is advisable to follow the order of the work as it is presented here when doing the program for the first time. Once you are familiar with all the exercises, movements and elongations, work out a routine best suitable for yourself. You can be selective and choose to work with some parts of the program that you believe will benefit you most.

If you are a health coach or a personal trainer working with clients, ask the client what part of the body they are most concerned about and start with selected exercises, using your intuition as a guide. Beginning with the clients' preferences makes for smooth energy flow. The more familiar you are with your client and the more familiar you become with the QBSc work, the more you can personalize your sessions, following your intuition. It is a good idea to keep up a conversation with your client. Speak just a bit more slowly than usual, in low tones. Ask for feedback. Does the client feel the energy? Keep her involved.

Preparing for body sculpting

There are several ways to prepare before starting a Body Sculpting program. I recommend you play around with all three options explained below. Try all three options, and adopt any or a combination of them as a way to move into a new way of wellbeing.

Getting in tune with the Life Force Energy

Before starting a Quantum Body Sculpting session take a few moments to go to your quiet space and 'turn on' the energy. Use either one of the three methods explained above or your own favorite method, to connect with the Life Force Energy: a. meditation combined with intention, b. Quantum Touch 'sweep and breathe' technique, c. The Shamanic Earth-Star meditation. Allow the energy to flow through your body. Imagine it. Feel it. And make it real.

Become fluid and flexible with laughter

To have a level of success in body sculpting one needs to be open-minded, flexible and willing to be true to oneself. Think of the way you feel when laughing. Try laugh for a few minutes every day, just for the fun of it. Laugh out loud for two minutes before starting the QBSc exercises. Your body will immediately begin to feel more relaxed, more fluid, more flexible. When laughing you somehow instantly become free of worries, expectations and hang-ups. Your endocrine system starts to produce endorphins, the marvelously powerful hormones that inhibit the transmission of painfully stressed feelings and create feelings of euphoria.

Have a beginners state of mind

To get the most out of a QBSc session, you need to have a beginner's state of mind, similar to the mind of a toddler, free of all expectations, ready to try anything that could be fun to do. Willing to have a good laugh at yourself even if you completely muff it. No worries, just keep on doing it for the beauty and the fun of it all. Do it, just because it feels good to do.

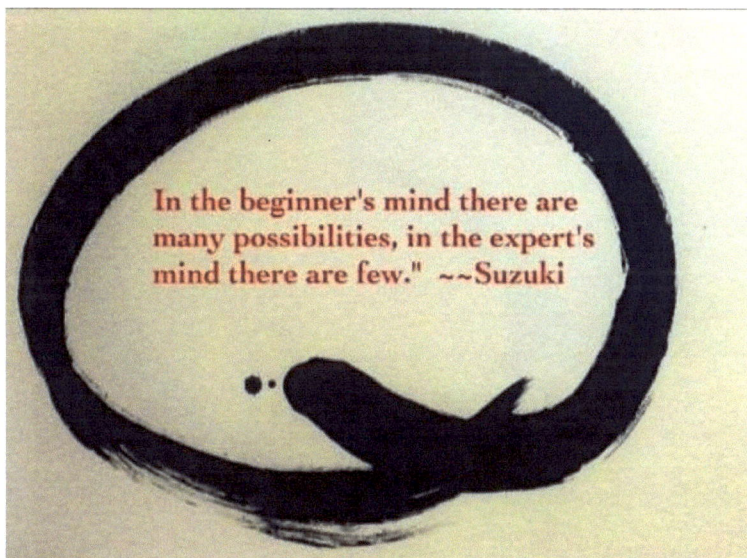

In the beginner's mind there are many possibilities, in the expert's mind there are few." ~~Suzuki

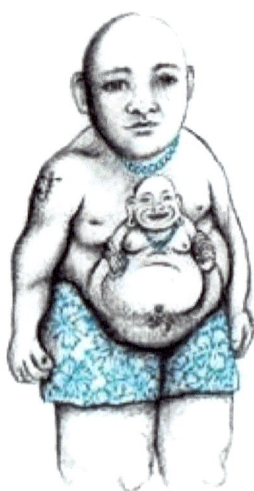

The Buddah didn't have to be thin to be popular!

The Buddha did not have to be thin to be popular

Meditation

I want to talk about using meditation and intention as a way to connect to the Life Force Energy. Let me share with you a primary method I use for regular meditation. If you regularly practice meditation, you may want to skip over this part, or simply skim read it to see if you agree. If you are not used to meditating, please try it. Imagine you are in a quiet spot where you will not be interrupted for a half-hour or more. Sit comfortably.

Remember, a lotus position is not required, especially not for people who do not have the physical ability to sit this way for an extended period. Breathe a little more slowly than normal and find your quiet place inside. Breathe in through the nose, and breathe out through slightly open lips. Imagine your breath goes in and out through your heart. Pay attention to the rhythm of your breathing and follow the up and down movements the breath creates on your abdomen. Pay attention to feeling the breath going in through your nose, and out over your lower lip. If external thoughts come in, acknowledge them and let them go. Say to yourself: "OK, I'm thinking about that now. It can wait till later," and focus your attention on your breathing again. Once you begin to feel more relaxed, find your place of highest focus. Internally say to yourself, "It is my intention to be in touch with the Life Force Energy." Pay attention to how your body feels. You may feel a warming sensation all over. You may feel a slight tingling sensation. You may feel nothing at all. With some practice, you will learn to go through these steps in less than a minute. You will very likely begin to have a sense of connectedness with all that is.

Not all meditators use the same breathing patterns. There are advantages to both breathing in through the nose and out through the mouth as well as there are advantages to breathing in and out through the nose. If you are new to meditation, it may be easier to create an awareness of your breath when breathing out through slightly pursed lips. In most of the exercises below, I recommend breathing in and out through the nose. Nasal breathing is slower than mouth breathing, and by slowing down the out-breath, the lungs have more time to extract oxygen from the air, a definite health benefit. I invite you to explore the different ways to find what is best for you. You can read more about different breathing techniques in my book 'Come Breathe With Us.'

A few moments of meditation are a right way to start a QBSc session.

Below is the text for a guided self-care meditation written for use when engaging in a Body Sculpting program. You can find a link to a recording with Binaural music background on our website: www.IEHealers.com. Alternatively, you may want to record the meditation in your own voice over the music of your choice. I recommend you listen to this recording repeatedly to boost your Body Sculpting progress.

A self-care meditation

A large part of the QBSc program involves being relaxed and at ease. Sculpting your body, first of all, means relaxing your body. The following brief self-care meditation has the intent to do just that.

Sit in a comfortable position facing a pleasing picture on your wall.
Imagine you are in one of your favorite places.
Close your eyes and breathe a little more slowly than normal. Imagine your breath goes in and out through your heart.
Bring your focus to behind your eyes.
Place your hands palms upward with thumb and ring finger touching.
Allow your body to relax. Breathe in through your heart, enjoy the inhale, and keep your focus behind your eyes. Breathe out through your heart. Slow down the exhale. Repeat this four times.

Open your eyes and look at the pleasing picture on the wall in front of you. Smile.

You are now ready to take back your power to care for yourselves and set your intentions to take responsibility for your well being.

Close your eyes again and as you do so allow your body to relax even more. Breathe.
Draw your attention to the shape of your body.
Maintain your smile. Feel your smile.
Imagine your body youth-full, relaxed, full of energy and vibrant.
Imagine it.   See it.   Feel it, and,   Make it real.

Every cell in your body is singing, dancing and smiling.
Join in with the singing. Enjoy the dancing. Feel that smile.
Breathe in the energy. Breathe out and let go of all imperfections in your body.
Breathe in youthfulness and while you breathe out let go of all age-related issues in your body.
Continue doing this for a few minutes.
When you are ready, slowly open your eyes and look at the pleasing picture on the wall in front of you.
Smile,
Be Youthful,   Be Well,   Be You.
And go on with the rest of your day.

Meditative breathing

Breathing, we all do it, but we do not all do it the same way. Many if not all healing modalities, yoga practices, and exercise programs I am familiar with place a lot of emphasis on the way to breathe properly. The meditative breathing method used in QBSc is my particular blend of techniques I have learned. People who are familiar with Core Breathing as taught by Alain Herriott will see some similarities to it. There also are overtones of Mental-physical breathing techniques. The very phrase I often use 'Breathe a little more slowly than normal' I borrowed from material taught by the Institute of HeartMath. While you are breathing slowly, focus on your heart space, as if your breath is going in and out through your heart. Recently, when reading Dr. Joe Dispenza's book 'Becoming Supernatural', I learned about a scientific explanation of his breathing techniques and saw definite similarities to what I have started to call 'Meditative Breathing.'

We do all the QBSc work using meditative breathing. Breathe in and out through the nose. Both the in and the out breath are equally important; the focus is a slow and regulated breathing rhythm. The rate and speed of your breathing need to be relaxed. Imagine your breath is going in and out through your heart. Always enjoy the inhale and prolong the exhale. During the inhale, tighten all the muscles of the abdominal floor, the PC muscles, and the lower abdominal muscles. Focus your thoughts on the area deep inside the top of your head. At the end of the inhale, keep the abdominal muscles tight and hold your breath for the count of 5. The exhale is controlled, relaxed and very slow. It is good to practice breathing this way for a while before starting the exercises so you can be comfortable doing them. Pay attention to how your body feels. How slow can you breathe while remaining relaxed? Try it, now and then.

Meditative breathing with Intent

Be Yourself

Meditative breathing with intent is a unique breathing pattern to help you to become quiet. It has an actively meditative focus with the intention of healing and shaping our body. It's a way to go to the heart of wellbeing at all levels of one's life. It is a way to experiment and to allow entrainment to a new level of being well.

"Be Yourself. Go deeper into who you really are."

Do the following brief meditation for a few minutes before you read on. Start by breathing slowly. Imagine your breath goes in and out through your heart. When you have reached your quiet place, set your intention. Say to your self: "It is my intention to be myself. It is my intention to go deeper into who I really am." Continue to breathe slowly for two minutes. Then ask yourself these three questions.

- Who am I, really?
- What am I?
- How deep am I able to allow myself to entrain to a new way of being?

Continue breathing slowly for another two minutes. Feel the awe and let in the quiet, entrain to your true self. Send heart love and energy to yourself.

Allowing

One of the fundamental concepts in the body sculpting program is 'allowing.' A dictionary defines the word allow as: "Let, permit, grant or concede the right for someone to do something." **Allow** implies the complete absence of an attempt, or even an intent, to hinder. Allowing, then, is like being in a state of free flow, which creates maximum flexibility and prepares one to be open to whatever will occur. Concerning body sculpting allowing means, we are holding the intent to allow the body to become well - proportioned. We are creating a state of openness using meditative breathing techniques. All the time we are free of attachment to the outcome or the unfolding of the process. We do have expectations and we let go of the result. Even though these thoughts may seem to be contradictory, they do belong. We do hold space for positive results and are open to surprises.

Earth - Star - Heart Meditation

There are many versions of the traditional Shamanic Earth - Star meditation. In my variation of a Shamanic Earth - Star meditation I add the heart connection. You can do this meditation anytime you wish. I advise you to end your Body Sculpting sessions with it. You can do the meditation in the privacy of your own home, in a park, or at a beach. You can imagine you are at your favorite place in nature.

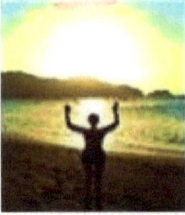

The meditation is available at www.IEHealers.com. Here follows the full text. You can also read it out loud and record it in your own voice for future use. In that case, speak in the first person singular. Start the recording with: "I invite the energies of Father Sky..." and so on. Speak slowly, allowing pauses between phrases. You can memorize the text and then personalize it.

It is a standing meditation. Stand comfortably with your feet just a bit more than shoulder-width apart. Your knees relaxed, but not bent. When doing the meditation as a group, make sure there is sufficient space between you and the persons next to you so you can freely move your arms. Breathe a little more slowly than normal. You can do this with your eyes open or closed. Stand relaxed. Raise your arms with palms facing upward. Focus your thoughts on a favorite star, on the heavens or the Divine.

Invite the energies of Father Sky to enter into your being, through the palms of your hands,

through the crown of your head,

and through every pore of your skin.

Allow the sensations to flow through your body.

Now bring your arms down with palms facing towards the earth. Focus your thoughts down into the center of the earth and invite the energy of Mother Earth to enter into your being,

58

through the palms of your hands,
through the soles of your feet,
and through every pore of your skin.
Invite the energies of the skies and the energies of the
earth to blend in your heart space and amplify them with
the love of your heart.
Allow those vibrations to reverberate within you for a
minute or two.
Bring your focus to your body,
to the skin on your neck and face,
to your shoulders
and to your back,
to your arms and legs
and to your entire body.
Allow yourself to relax.
You will likely have started to sway a bit. That's normal,
and that's good.
Pay attention to how your body feels. What you sense is
the energy of the Life Force vibrating within you. Allow it to
sculpt you and allow it make you feel and be well. When
you are ready, please sit down and take in your
surroundings. Commit yourself to allow the Life Force
Energy to assist you:
to be healthy and well,
to be well proportioned,
to be beautiful,
to be you.

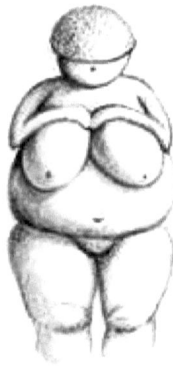

The Venus of Willendorf discovered in 1908 in Austria is said to be over 25,000 years old - probably the oldest example of mother Goddess

Intention

Intention and energy healing go hand in hand. The breathing techniques used in energy healing bring about quiet vibrations to the heart, the brain, and the mind. When there is coherence between the heart and the mind we are in a state where healing can happen in the body. In such a state of heart-brain coherence, intentions become a tremendously powerful and useful tool to manifest your desires.

The heart and essence of Quantum Body Sculpting are using energy and sending the vibrations of love from the heart to the body. We set an intention for the body to heal, to find its way back to pristine health, having an anatomically correct and a proportionally pleasing shape.

Lynne McTaggart in her book 'The Intention Experiment' explains the Intention technique in some detail. She calls it Powering Up.

Allow me to take you through my version of an Intention exercise.

61

Please sit comfortably and close your eyes. Breathe a little more slowly than normal. Place your focus behind your eyes. Now drop into your heart space. Internally repeat: "It is my intention to feel relaxed, refreshed, and youthful for the rest of the evening, for tomorrow, and for the rest of the weekend. From then on I intend to be able to recall the feeling of being relaxed and youthful and emit those vibrations to my appearance." Hold that thought for a full two minutes, in silence. At any time you remember setting this intention right here and at this time, you will be able to recall the vibrations you are experiencing now.

Your thoughts have a definite impact. When setting an intention, you need to align your intention with the desired outcome. You need to have a clear and confident desire. Focus on a positive result. Have and hold a pure and positive emotional attitude. It all makes a difference in the outcome of your intention.

Getting to Know Your Body

The 5 Diaphragms

Many people know about the importance of breathing from the diaphragm. We think of the large muscle at the top of the abdomen when talking about the diaphragm. It is known as the Peritoneum diaphragm. Since learning more about alternative healing, I have become aware that we have five diaphragms. In yoga literature, I have read about three diaphragms, referred to as the respiratory, pelvic, and laryngeal diaphragms. Some craniosacral sources I have read cite four. In the International Journal of Complementary & Alternative Medicine five diaphragms are discussed. It becomes confusing when different names appear for the same diaphragms. What's been more important to me is becoming aware of the five diaphragms as areas whose release causes larger areas of the body to be affected. I have learned to release my diaphragms. Releasing the diaphragms has made noticeable positive

63

results to my overall health. I also has improved my posture.

The more commonly known peritoneum diaphragm is the one associated with the lungs. But all five diaphragms are influenced by the act of breathing and hence are affected by the movements of our main anatomical diaphragm.

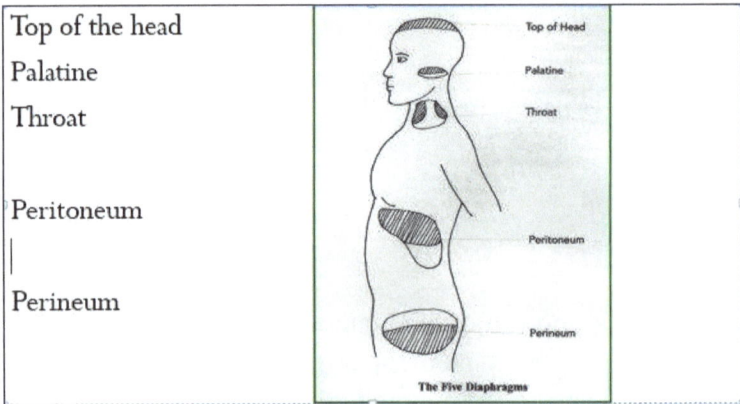

Top of the head	Top of Head
Palatine	Palatine
Throat	Throat
Peritoneum	Peritoneum
Perineum	Perineum

The Five Diaphragms

Following are examples of the sensations produced when the tension in the muscles of the diaphragms and surrounding areas is released.

1. The Peritoneum Diaphragm

The peritoneum diaphragm is a multilayered membrane or muscle lining the abdominal cavity which supports and covers the organs within it. The exercise that follows covers the entire torso. You're likely to feel it most readily in the kidney region. Your kidneys are located in the middle of the back towards the bottom of the ribcage. The sensation that you will likely feel is one of softening. The feeling may continue up through the ribcage and down through the lower back as well as spread throughout the entire abdomen. It will feel as if your back has a warm flowing relaxation moving through it.

2. Throat diaphragm

The area affected by the throat diaphragm runs from the first rib up into the lower jaw. When putting your attention on it, you may feel as if your whole neck expands and softens. Initially, you may sense a slight buzzing around the Adam's Apple area. Eventually, you will feel relaxation through the entire area. One side effect of releasing the throat area is an increase of salivation and the teeth in the lower jaw may relax and even align some.

3. The Perineum Diaphragm

The Perineum diaphragm area is between the genitals and the anus in both males and females. It covers the surface area from the pubic bone to the tailbone. It supports the entire pelvic floor. The muscles are diamond shaped. When the diaphragm is relaxed it feels like a dome and a warming sensation rises and elongates throughout the pelvic floor all the way up through the hips. It releases the surface area to about an inch or two into the body cavities.

4. The Crown Diaphragm

The crown diaphragm is located at the top of the head. Releasing it affects the entire scalp as well as the cranial sutures. It may feel as if the top of the head is opening up.

You may have a sensation of a crawling feeling on top of the scalp, or as if a light cap on the head is lifting or expanding.

5. The Palatine Diaphragm

The palatine diaphragm is located at the level of the upper palate. It has an irregularly shaped bone which forms part of the nasal cavity. It articulates with six bones: the sphenoid, ethmoid, maxilla inferior nasal concha, vomer and the opposite palatine. Because it interacts with all these bones, it affects the entire upper portion of the skull as well as the upper jaw on both sides of the head and into the base of the brainpan and sinus cavity. When releasing this area it may feel as if your sinuses are opening and as if there is more space in your mouth and jaw. The release of tensions in this diaphragm may align teeth and ease TMJ issues. The release of the palatine diaphragm causes flexion of the sphenoid bone creating more space for the brain.
If you hold your finger right next to and in front of the ear cavity you will feel where your jaw hinges. It gives you a good idea where this area starts.

When doing the exercises with the diaphragms, a light touch of each of the areas of the individual diaphragms is likely to raise your awareness of these áreas. It will usually expand your awareness of larger areas around them as well. As you learn to increase an awareness of the regions affected by each of the five diaphragms, one at the time, you may be able to learn to sense all simultaneously as you do meditative breathing. It may take some practice. ☺

The 5 Diaphragm Exercises

The exercises that follow build on each other. Be sure to take your time and become comfortable with the activities. Allow yourself to fully experience how each practice unfolds. Everyone's body will absorb the benefits in its own unique manner. It's about everyone's personal development, enjoy. You may become aware of what seems like incredibly small changes are happening. Nevertheless, you will be able to affect changes on a profound level. You will learn to isolate specific muscles, tendons, and bones in almost any part of your anatomy. Some precise anatomical terminology will help you get it right.

It may take some practice for you to become sensitive at this level we are dealing with the body. Knowing what is inside the areas you are focusing on, often makes it easier to release tensions. When tensions are released, your body shape improves. We do each exercise with the Meditative Breath. Your focus needs to stay behind the eyes and at the same time your peripheral attention needs to be in the area you are releasing. Your attention goes there, but you need not look there. As an example: you need not look at your foot to know that you are wiggling your toes.

Depending on the amount of guarding you have in an area you may have a bit of difficulty to sense anything. The guarding may not allow you to feel safe to feel anything there at all. Such blocks may have been created by any event from the past, such as an injury, or by verbal or physical abuse, or as a result of a limiting belief system or Victorian upbringing. Beginning with practicing feeling sensations in a relatively 'easy to sense' area may help with allowing access in more guarded areas. You will feel newly released areas readily integrate with the rest of the body.

Recall the 'sweep and breathe' exercises we use to get connected to the Life Force Energy. They are a teaching tool, from the feather's slight touch to a small brush with an imaginary feather, to bring about body awareness and the sensation of feeling the energy. Similarly, the slight stroking of the areas of the five diaphragms needs to be a very light touch. You do not have to continue it once you learn to be aware of the sensations that meditative breathing creates in these areas.

Do not set unrealistic expectations for yourself of what you will be able to sense. Everyone's journey through their body is unique.

For each of the following five exercises lie down on your back on a yoga mat. Flat on your back with your arms at your side and your knees slightly bent.

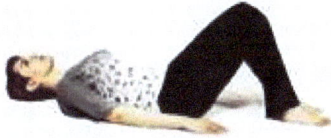

1. Breathe several meditative breaths. Hold your breath for a few moments at the end of each breath.
Very lightly stroke the perineal floor or the outside of your hips at the area of your crotch.
Exhale, keep your focus inside your head behind the eyes and note any sensation in this area.

2. Breathe several meditative breaths in this position on the yoga mat. Hold your breath for a few moments at the end of each breath.
Lightly stroke the sides of your body at the level of the kidneys.
Exhale, keep your focus inside your head behind the eyes and note any sensation in this area.

3. Breathe several meditative breaths in this position on the yoga mat. Hold your breath at the end of each breath.
Very lightly stroke your neck near your Adam's apple.
Exhale, keep your focus inside your head behind the eyes and note any sensation in this area.

4. Breathe several meditative breaths in this position on the yoga mat. Hold your breath at the end of each breath.
Stroke both sides of your face right in front of the ear canals.
Exhale, keep your focus inside your head behind the eyes and note any sensation in this area.

5. Breathe several meditative breaths in this position on the yoga mat. Hold your breath at the end of each breath.
Stroke the top of your head or your hair or just above our head.
Exhale, keep your focus inside your head behind the eyes and note any sensation in this area.

Alternate Ways to Release the 5 Diaphragms

Visualize the area of one of the diaphragms in your mind's eye while doing Meditative Breathing.
Try relaxing the area on the inhale. Hold your breath for the count of 5. Exhale slowly, take a break and repeat with your focus on the next diaphragm. Spend 15 to 20 minutes focusing on the different diaphragms.
Be ready to sense subtle changes happening in any or all five areas, one after another, creating a wave.
Experiment with releasing tension in any areas of your body.

Benefits of Releasing Tension in the Five Diaphragms

Perineum Diaphragm

In men, learning to release the perineum diaphragm will bring relief of prostate problems. In women, it may result in more relaxed or less painful menstrual cycles. For both women and men being able to release the perineum diaphragm results in increased sexual satisfaction.

Peritoneum Diaphragm

The more we can release the main diaphragm, the easier it becomes to do deep breathing. Releasing the diaphragm brings about a simultaneous release of tensions in the solar plexus. People with a relaxed peritoneum diaphragm usually are free of lower back tensions.

Throat Diaphragm

Releasing the throat diaphragm brings about a release in all of the neck area, the upper back and shoulders. It will resolve the tension in the brachial plexus, the nerve fibers running from the spine through the neck, the armpits, and the arms. Frequently, long-standing neck pain disappears.

71

Palatine Diaphragm

With a released palatine diaphragm tension in the skull will lessen. It will make it easier to breathe through the nose, and provide relief of sinus issues. You will also have more flexion of the sphenoid bone.

Crown Diaphragm

A more flexible crown diaphragm will sometimes give spontaneous release of cranial sutures. It will provide a reduction in headaches. In general, it will improve the energy flow through your body.

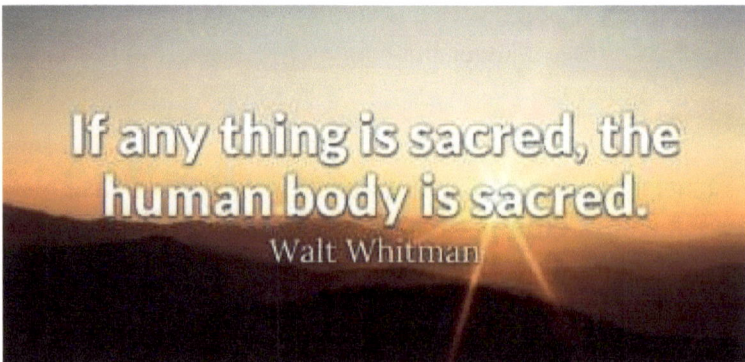

If any thing is sacred, the human body is sacred.
Walt Whitman

Movements and Elongations

Our bodies are a dynamic entity ready and open to the flow of energy. In the exercises that follow, the moves engage the bones and joints. Make all movements during the out-breath only. During the outbreath, our muscles relax, and change is smooth. Ergo, moving on the outbreath is less likely to cause injury. Do every exercise while doing the Meditative Breath. Breathe a little more slowly than normal. Tighten your PC and lower abdominal muscles and follow your in-breath as if it starts in your abdomen, using the peritorium diaphragm. From there imagine that your breath flows through your heart space and towards the top of your head. Your focus needs to follow your breath, and at the same time, your peripheral attention needs to be in the area you are releasing. All breathing is through the nose. During any exercise or movement keep your focus inside the top of your head, behind your eyes. The exercises are like 'speed bumps' to assist you in slowing down. Ask yourself the question:

"Can I move 'like this' and maintain a sense of openness?"
Approach each exercise with an opening for new possibilities. Becoming quiet inside is key in body sculpting. It helps to have a child-like attitude and an openness to evolve.

A few comments about elongating as compared to stretching. Allow me to define the words.
An elongation is a slow movement to lengthen, with the intention to create and maintain greater length and reduce width.
A stretch is a movement to lengthen temporarily, with the expectation that the object has enough elasticity to go back to the previous size.
Elongating your muscles allows your joints to move through their entire ranges of motion. It gives you freedom of movement and eliminates tightness that can hamper performance and lead to injury.
When you elongate, 'the action pulls on the fibers within your muscles, reducing the amount of overlap that is present in the thin and thick muscle fibers when your muscles are at rest. Whether you elongate or stretch out your muscle fibers, it activates a stretch reflex, which is your body's way of preventing you from elongating your muscles too much and causing injury. '
cf. 4929.html https://healthyliving.azcentral.com/stretching-elongate-muscles-
The slower the movement, the less of a stretch reflex occurs. When practicing Body Sculpting, you set your intention to elongate, not to stretch.
In addition to elongating muscles, the movements also increase blood flow to your muscles. It is beneficial

because your muscles need oxygen to function, and blood cells bring oxygen to your muscles. Performing elongations may also help you increase your strength when lifting weights and improve your endurance when performing any cardiovascular activity.

The exercises are in a particular order and build on each other. It is essential to take your time to experience how each practice unfolds. Everyone's body will unfold in its unique manner. There's no need to be overly ambitious. It is all about everyone's personal development. You may become aware that incredibly small changes are happening. Because of this, you will be able to affect changes on a deep level. You will learn to isolate specific muscles, tendons, and bones, almost any part of your anatomy. Some rather specific anatomical terminology is used to help with this. It may take some practice to become sensitive at this level, but it **will** happen and knowing what is inside the areas of your body you are focusing on, often makes it easier to release tensions. Go ahead and read some pages on the human anatomy online in your spare time to get on a first name basis with the organs, muscles, and bones in your body. It is good to get to know yourself inside and out.

Sensing the Support of the Earth

The first exercise, known as a ground scan, is an awareness exercise. We are scanning our bodies to increase our awareness of where our body's tensions are located. This awareness is to be used as a baseline to compare with after each of the exercises that follow. This first exercise is referred to as a ground scan throughout the rest of the practices.

After doing the ground scan, as well as after doing any of the other exercises, it is essential to allow your body a few moments to assimilate any changes that have happened. Ground scans need to be done on a firm surface, a yoga mat or a regular carpet. Repeating the ground scan after doing any other exercise will also allow you to sense any changes that may have happened.

The purpose of the ground scan is to get a sense of what parts of your body touch the earth when lying down, and how you allow the earth to support you.

The benefit is developing an openness to new possibilities of interacting with the earth, and with the universe as a whole.

Before doing the ground scan, set the following intention. "It is my intention to be completely relaxed and at ease, while doing a ground scan."

You can say any or all of the following positive affirmations, or make up similar statements of your own.

"I feel comfortable with myself."

76

"I trust the earth to support me."
"I am safe and at ease in this position."

The exercise

Lie on your back, with your arms relaxed at your side, your legs outstretched, and your feet hip-width apart.

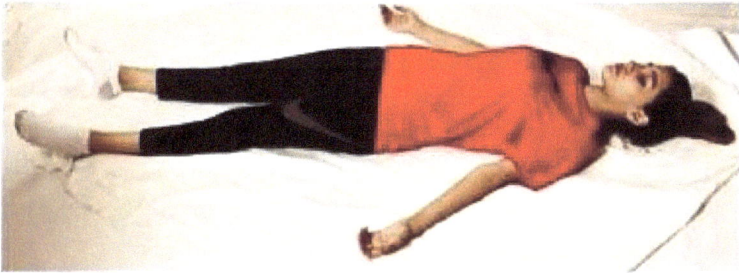

Feel where each part of your body is touching the ground. Notice the areas where your body does not touch the ground. How big are they? Answer the question in detail. What fits through there: a mouse, a cat, an elephant ☺. Be imaginative, not realistic. Do not measure, just get a feel for it.

What parts of your body resist being supported or touched?
Pay attention to your neck, your ankles, your lower back, back of your knees, shoulders, wrists, and your fingers. Breathe into all the places where your body touches the earth.

Notice any tension and the amount of space. Use this awareness as a baseline to compare with after doing the following exercises.

When finished, walk around a few steps and try a different point of view.
Again, lie on your back, arms relaxed at your side, legs outstretched, and your feet hip-width apart.

Is there a place where you want a pillow? BUT DO NOT PUT A PILLOW THERE! Why would you want support there? What if there were no pillows? How can your body, your mind, your intentions accommodate to give you the support you need? Ask your body to find a way to become comfortable with the earth you are resting on, without any props or pillows. Breathe into any areas of tension.
How does the earth support you? Are you allowing the earth to support you? What parts of your body do not require support? Is the support you feel evenly distributed among the various places the earth supports you? Do you feel safe with the earth's support?
When you have completed the exercise, take a moment to re-read the questions and reflect on your answers. Write down your impressions to refer back to a week and a month later when doing the exercise again. Has anything changed?

Use this awareness as a baseline and to compare with after doing the exercises.

Anchored-Sacrum Exercise

When you do the anchored sacrum exercise, move slowly. Pretend someone is pulling up your leg at the kneecap. Remember to move only on the out-breath. Each time you need to take a new breath, stop all movements and continue the movement on the next out-breath. When the upward movement of your legs is complete, your knees are bent, your heels as close to the body as possible while remaining comfortable, and your feet are flat on the floor. No particular distance in motion is required, you are not looking for perfection.

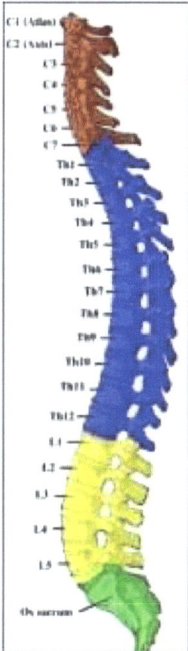

After completing the exercise rest a bit and drink some water. If lying on the floor is difficult the exercise can be done on a massage table, or similar firm surface, but not on a soft mattress.

The purpose of the exercise is to create an awareness of the energy flow in your body in two directions, from the sacrum downwards and out the feet, and from the lowest vertebra of your lower back, L5, upwards and out the top of your head.

The benefit of this exercise is increased blood flow to your legs and feet. Also, your posture will improve.

Set your intention internally before starting the exercise, saying: "It is my intention to gain awareness of the movement of energy in my body."

While doing the exercise, you can use these positive affirmations.
"My energy is flowing through my body."
"I am healthy and well."
"I love it how I can feel my energy moving."

The exercise

Begin with a ground scan. Lie down with your arms at your side and your feet no wider than hip-width apart. Begin meditative breathing.

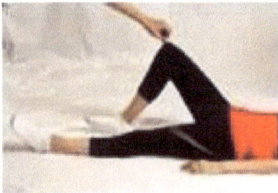

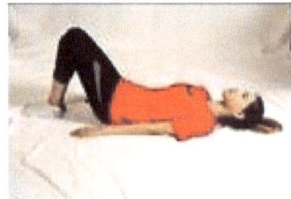

Bring your knees up, one at the time, moving only on the exhale. Move slowly, as if someone is pulling up your leg at the kneecap. When the upward movement is complete your knees are bent, your heels as close to the body as possible, and your feet flat on the floor.
Imagine your sacrum is solidly glued to the ground.
On each exhale sense the flow of energy in two directions. Bring your legs down, one at the time, with your heels leading and your toes back.

Come to a sitting position, breathe, and then come to a to a standing position. Walk around slowly and notice any changes in your posture and movement.

Elongations with a Towel

Do the exercises without wearing shoes. Fold a bath towel length-wise and roll it firmly to make a roll of about 10 – 15 centimeters in diameter and the width of your back. When you are uncomfortable in a position, you may unroll the towel to the correct size. These are four separate exercises, each with a towel in a different position.

Here are some hints and possible difficulties you may encounter. In position A, if your chin is putting pressure on your chest, unroll the towel a bit to be more comfortable. In position B, with a towel under the neck, your head is suspended, and you should feel traction in your neck. The towel needs to be snug to your shoulders, and your head should not touch the floor. If the position is not comfortable, you can adjust the towel.
In position C, if your hands remain hanging in mid-air, use a pillow to support your forearms, or rest your hands on your torso.
In position D, you can adjust the towel size if necessary. There should be no pressure on your tailbone. It should feel as if your lower back is being gently rounded down and opened up.

Between each position do a ground scan and feel if there are any changes, however subtle. Pay attention to how your body holds tensions and how it releases them.
Each position should take about 5 minutes, for a total of about 20 minutes. Once you feel the energy continuously flowing through your body, the exercise is complete. When you are ready, walk around a bit and pay attention if you sense any changes in the way you move. Remember to take a drink of water after each exercise.

The purpose of the following exercises is to create space and elongate the body. It will alert you to sense any irregularities in your body. Placing a towel in the way changes the way we relate to feeling the energy flow.

The benefit is getting an increased awareness of the existence of any blockages in your energy flow. The exercise makes it easier to sense 'speed bumps' in the energy flow. Once we can sense artificial 'bumps' or blockages, we will know what to look for and how to identify existing blockages in our system. For practitioners and massage therapists, once you learn to recognize blockages in your energy flow, you also can learn to become sensitive to blockages in the energy flow of your clients.

Internally set your intention by saying,"It is my intention to release all blockages."

During the exercise repeat some positive affirmations. Here are some examples.
"It's great to know the limitations and potentials of my body."

"I am open to moving on to new possibilities of greater wellness."

The exercises

Do a ground scan. Take note of your energy flow to compare it with after doing the exercises. Begin meditative breathing. On the exhale raise your knees, one at a time, dragging your heels.

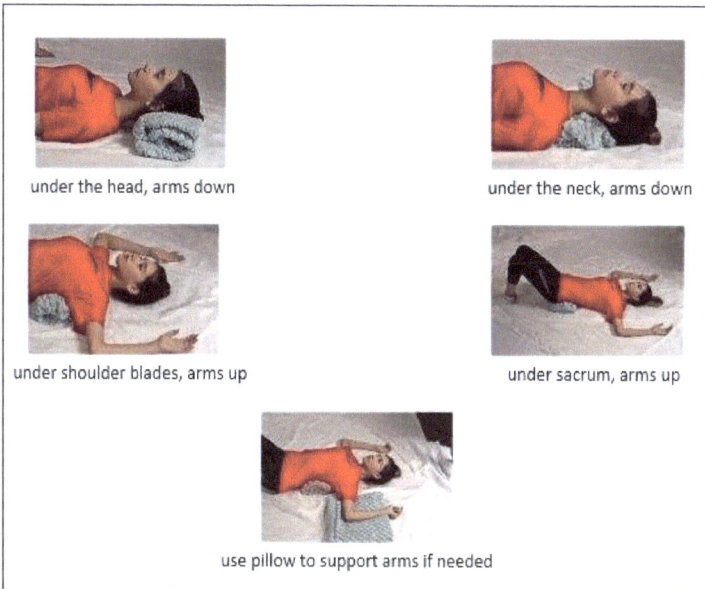

under the head, arms down

under the neck, arms down

under shoulder blades, arms up

under sacrum, arms up

use pillow to support arms if needed

When both your knees are up, place the towel in the positions shown in the diagram. Rest your arms on the side of your body for exercises A and B. For exercises C and D place your arms in a stick-up position as shown. Find the wave your breath creates from the sacrum to the crown and beyond. Continue meditative breathing for a few

83

minutes. Sense how you are holding yourself. Are you bracing or allowing? Breathe into any areas of tension until you sense your body has released all the tension it can do for now. Remove the towel, bring your legs down one at a time. Remember to move on the out-breath only. Lead with your heels and keep your toes pointed towards you. Elongate your body by imagining you are pushing a heavy object along the floor with your feet, moving it as far away from you as possible.

Once you feel the energy continuously flowing through your body, each exercise is complete. Walk around a bit and pay attention if there are any changes in the way you move. Remember to drink water after each practice. Do a ground scan after each position and ask yourself if the exercise has affected how the earth supports you.

Standing Elongation

The standing elongation exercise happens mainly in your imagination. The few steps walking are for real. Before starting the exercise review the notes on the five diaphragms.

The purpose of the exercise is to create awareness of any limitations your body has, in particular concerning your posture.
The benefit of repeating this exercise frequently and regularly is that it will help you to stand tall and walk to elongate your spine.
Internally set your intention by saying:
"It is my intention that I at all times stand tall and walk with ease."
During the exercise repeat some positive affirmations.
Here are some examples.
"I walk tall at all times."
"My spine is upright and has an anatomically correct curvature."
"I love my posture."

The exercise

Stand tall, with your feet shoulder-width apart. Tie an imaginary 100-pound weight to the bottom of your sacrum. Create awareness through all five diaphragms while walking a few steps with the load on the sacrum. Walk slowly and feel the weight.

Now attach the top of your head to a bungee cord attached to an imaginary ceiling five feet above your head. In your imagination allow your body to grow taller, to elongate. (not stretch!) Walk a few steps this way.

Breathe into any areas where you experience any tension, whether imaginary or real. Become aware of any limitations your body senses, and move on from that awareness to new possibilities.

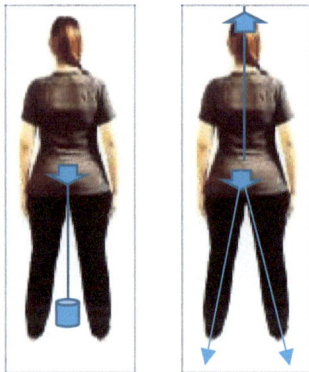

In picture 1 the sacrum feels as if a 100 pounds weight is hanging from it, pulling it down. In picture 2 sense a wave through the body out the top of the head and down through the legs and the feet.

Standing Knee Bend Elongation

Even doing the exercise only once is likely to improve your gait. Repetition on a regular basis will bring about a more relaxed way of walking. To read more detailed explanations of the exercise look up the Feldenkrais method.

It is essential to keep your neck angled slightly downward and relaxed throughout the exercise.

Pay attention to how the Meditative Breath feels and how bending the knees affects the energy flow in your body. Try to do it with a slight smile on your face. The exercise is done without shoes, standing on a yoga mat, or on a carpeted floor, or barefoot in the grass.

The purpose of this exercise is that it frees up the pelvis, the sacrum as well as the entire spine.

The benefit is that you will gain a better posture and will begin to walk with more ease.

Internally set your intention before starting the exercise by saying: "It is my intention that all the vertebrae in my back move with ease. It is my intention to walk with proper posture."

During the exercise repeat some positive affirmations. Here are some examples.

"I have great posture."

"I can move in any direction I want with ease and grace."

"My gait is graceful."

"I love the way I can move and the way I can walk."

The exercise

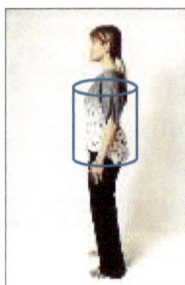

To start the exercise stand with your knees straight but not locked. Begin meditative breathing, and remember that all movements are done on the out-breath only. Imagine the trunk of your body is encaged in a large tube as shown in the picture. Be careful not to touch the tube when you move down and up. Bend your knees on the exhale until your kneecap hides your toes when you are looking down.

Stay put in this position and take a few breaths.
On the next exhale come up slowly. Your weight is mostly on your heels. If you feel your weight mainly on the ball of your feet, lean back a bit to shift your weight to your heels, and try the exercise again. You may feel a slight tension in the muscles in the backside of your calves and around your ankles.
Move very slowly.
Walk around a bit and pay attention to how it feels to walk after this exercise. You may feel subtle changes. Then again some changes may manifest a day or two later.

Walking

The way we walk tells a lot about us. When Everett, my husband, was in his mid-sixties I noticed he was beginning to walk just like his ten years older brother: Head forward, shoulders slumping and his butt sticking out backward. I used to slap him on the butt and say: "Try to walk straight." A few years later I taught a workshop I called 'Core and More' which included many QiGong exercises, including the walking exercise below. We practiced and practiced for me to perfect the movements with the intent to be able to teach them well. It improved Everett's gait. Everett is my editor and as such is going over the exercises in great detail. In his imagination, he is doing them all. It builds on the 'Core and More' work we did years ago. You should see his posture and his gait now. He moves as if he is ten years younger than 15 years ago.

I began to pay attention to the way people walk. I noticed people slumping at relatively young ages and those who stooped and slumped looked older to me, even when I knew their actual ages. When getting up from a chair, many people start with their heads moving forwards. Next, they lift their bodies from the chair or sofa by placing their hands on the seat or arms of the chair and pushing up with the muscles in their arms, only gradually straightening out over the first several steps, if at all.

The purpose of the exercise is to continue elongations and to reduce the amount of rigidity and tension in your torso and to learn to walk erect.

The benefit is learning to walk in a more centered way, to improve one's gait and look younger.

Internally set your intention by saying, "It is my intention to walk erect. It is my intention to look youthful when I walk." While doing the exercise repeat some positive affirmations. Here are some examples.

"I walk with ease and grace."

"I love my posture."

"I look youthful at all times."

The exercise

There are two parts to the walking exercise:

1. Extending through the body, one side at the time, and shuffling the feet.
2. Experiencing how to walk more efficiently, while moving from the sacrum. I now think of it as 'walking from the hips.'

Part 1. To begin the exercise stand with your feet hip-width apart. If your toes point out, widen your stance from your heels. Allow your arms to hang loosely at your sides, and keep your head and your neck relaxed. Begin meditative breathing and close your eyes. All movements again are done on the out-breath only and very slowly.

Do a grounding exercise by bringing your attention into the center of the earth. Imagine you are a tree, deeply rooted in the ground. Slowly raise your arms, and wave them as if they are the branches of a tree. Feel the strength of the tree and its relationship to the earth. Imagine yourself as

90

surely grounded as the tree. Internally thank Mother Earth for her support. Next bring your arms down to your sides again.

Now bring your feet close together, but not quite touching. Extend yourself with one leg, as if that leg is growing taller, and allow your torso on the same side to grow taller, or lengthen. This way you are lifting your weight off your other foot. Slide your other foot forward.

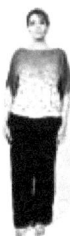

Now repeat the same movements on the other side and take four shuffle steps. Open your eyes, cease the meditative breathing, and gradually start walking faster. Allow your arms to move as they wish. Place one hand on your sacrum applying firm pressure as you walk around. The walking movement starts at your hips. Your torso, neck and head readily come along. Pay attention how it feels to walk this way.

Part 2 is an exercise in trust. Do not get overzealous. It takes some time and confidence to find a new center when walking. Work with a partner, a "driver". The partner's hand is on your sacrum. You lean (lightly) into your partner's hand. The "Driver" pushes you forward a few steps at a time.

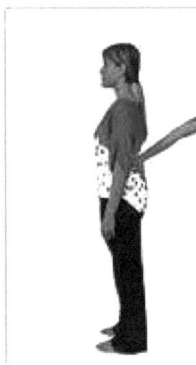

Be aware of the increased ease and flexibility in your lower back while walking. The driver's hand controls the speed and impetus to move. Walk around for a minute or two and change roles.

91

Bending Forward

In the forward bending exercise you will be releasing tension in the spine and creating more space between the vertebrae. It is likely you will learn a lot about the flows that move through your body and how to open and relax areas where you feel any tension. You will find your blockages and learn to release them. If at any given point during the exercise you sense a lot of tension building, stop a moment or two in that position and breathe into the area of stress. Allow the tension to release as much as possible. Continue the movement during the next out breath. It is of crucial importance to move VERY SLOWLY.

The intent of the forward-bend is not necessarily to touch the toes. The key is to follow the flow, and when you start to feel as if you are stressing, STOP. It does NOT matter how far down your fingertips can reach.

Imagine there are two pulleys in your back, while the body releases one vertebra at the time as you allow yourself to bend down. Next, reel in the pulleys one vertebra at the time when coming up again. Pulley # 1 is between the shoulder blades at the 6th thoracic vertebra (T6). Pulley # 2 is at the sacrum just above your hip bones.

Pay attention to the difference between the upper and the lower half of your body, above and below the sacrum. On the exhale, while connected to the flow of energy through the body, pull your navel to the spine to emphasize the division.

Stay 'in the moment.' Do not worry how far down you can bend. Notice how you feel and experience the release of each vertebra. Do the exercise carefully and very slowly. Stay with the meditative breath.

The purpose of the exercise is to continue elongations and to reduce the amount of rigidity and tension in the neck and head carriage. You will be releasing tension in the spine and creating room between the vertebrae.

The benefit is that you are learning to walk in a more centered way.

Internally set your intention by saying, "It is my intention to be as flexible as possible and appropriate for my body. It is my intention to be able to sense each of my vertebrae release, one at the time."

During the exercise repeat some positive affirmations. Here are some examples.
"I am relaxed and flexible."
"It is easy for me to bend."
"I love doing these exercises."

The exercise

Before starting the bending forward exercise do the Grounding exercise (the tree imagery explained above), feel the energy go through your body and out the top of your head. Start releasing the pulley between your shoulder blades and allow your head to slowly drop forward and down as far as it will go. Allow your hands and arms to hang loose. Only move on the exhale.

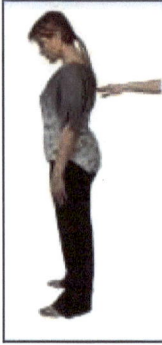

Move to the second pulley, start releasing the thoracic vertebrae from the top down, one at the time. Everything up from the last vertebra in your lower back (L5) lengthens.
Coming up, just reverse the process. With your awareness on the sacrum, reel in one vertebra at the time, from the bottom up. Once the shoulders are all the way back, begin reeling in with the first pulley and bring your head up to its normal position.

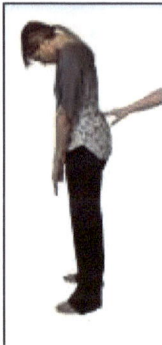

Walk around a few steps using your new awareness of walking from the hips. Pay attention to how your body feels.

94

Lifting and Loving your Breasts

Many women over 40 (and sometimes younger) tend to blame gravity and breastfeeding practices for sagging breasts. The prevalence of breast reduction, breast enlargement, and breast lift surgery suggests that women's concerns about breast size and shape are widespread. Statistics reported by various sources vary concerning the percentage of the women who are dissatisfied with their breasts. All stats I have seen indicate the percentage is well over 50%.

Younger and thinner women tend to be worried about their breasts being too small. Women of all ages worry about their breasts being too large. Older and heavier women seem to be more concerned about breast droopiness.

Massively oversized and sagging breasts may cause medical problems such as chronic pains to the head, neck and shoulders. Secondary health problems, such as poor blood circulation, impaired breathing, or chafing of the skin of the chest and the underside of the breasts may also occur. Then, there may be issues such as brassiere-strap indentations to the shoulders and the improperly fitting of clothing.

The medical industry offers cosmetic surgery as solutions for both breast enlargement and breast reduction. They include implants, lifts, surgery with or without liposuction.

95

All of these have non-beneficial side effects with varying degrees of seriousness.

The Qi Gong exercise we propose offers an alternative to creams and oils, pumps, pills, surgical lifts, and implants. We do not suggest that our technique can solve all breast related issues, but we do guarantee there are no adverse counter indications. Doing the exercise will improve the way you feel about your breasts and the way they look.

The purpose of this exercise is to improve the energy flow through the breast area, to lessen and remove any blockages from the lymph nodes and vessels, and to open lymphatic fluid pathways through the breasts. The movements will stimulate circulation, increase lymph flow and release stagnation at the cellular and tissue levels. The benefit of the exercise is the development of firm and shapely breasts. The exercise also is an excellent preventive measure for breast cancer and improves one's overall breast health.

Internally set your intention by saying:"It is my intention to have healthy and shapely breasts. It is my intention that my lymphatic system works at optimum capacity."
During the exercise repeat some positive affirmations.
Here are some examples. You can make up your own.
"I love the shape of my body."
"I have healthy breast tissue."
"I trust these exercises are good for me."
Make sure you keep the movements slow and smooth to allow for empowered lymph flow to take place.

The exercise

To begin the exercise start meditative breathing.

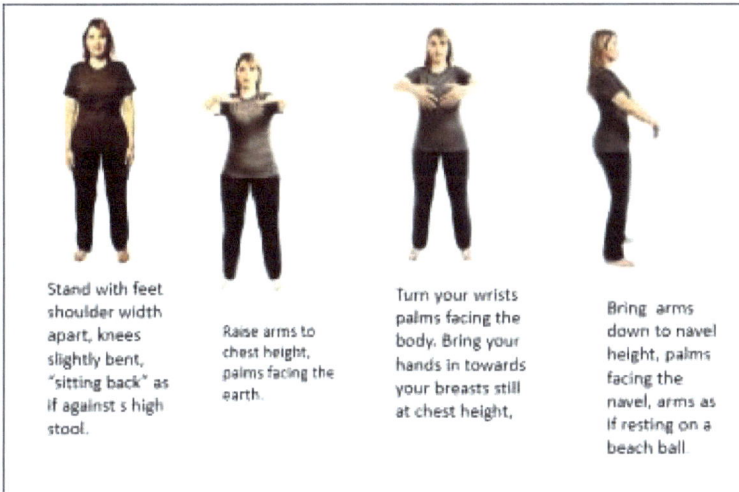

Stand with feet shoulder width apart, knees slightly bent, "sitting back" as if against s high stool.

Raise arms to chest height, palms facing the earth.

Turn your wrists palms facing the body. Bring your hands in towards your breasts still at chest height,

Bring arms down to navel height, palms facing the navel, arms as if resting on a beach ball.

1. Stand with your feet shoulder-width apart, your knees slightly bent. It feels like "sitting back" as if leaning against a high stool. Your arms are alongside your body. You are fully grounded.
2. Raise your arms to chest height with your palms facing the earth. You are bringing the earth's energy up.
3. Turn your wrists towards you and move them closer to your chest while raising your elbows out. Your arms are in a position as if you are hugging a tree. You are bringing the energy into your body.
4. Move your hands down to navel height. Your palms are now facing your navel. During this move, you are allowing the energy to travel through your core.

5. Turn your wrist to have your palms facing the earth again while moving your arms down. This way you are settling the energy.
6. Return your arms to be alongside your body again.
7. Repeat the exercise several times.

Be Free to Feel Young Again

Remember rolling in the grass as a child?

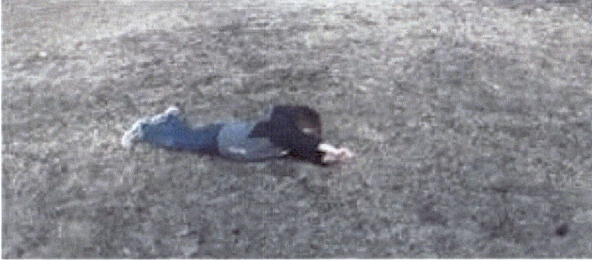

Today I invite to join in the fun as an adult.

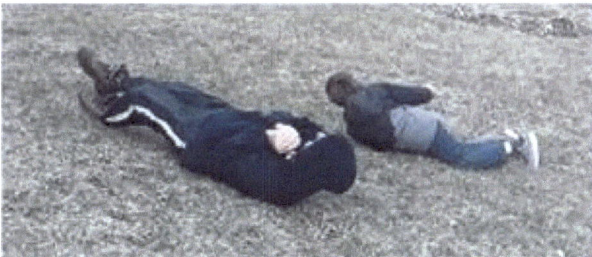

When I showed these pictures at the first QBSc workshop in Laredo Texas, the immediate answer to the invitation was an enthusiastic "Yes!"

We were in the presentation room at Bella's Beauty Salon on a busy Street in Laredo, Texas. There were no grassy fields or hillsides within a half hour commuting distance. Everyone pitched in to put chairs and tables aside, and we did the Lipo-roll on the tile floor. What fun! When at the end of the room someone shouted: "Let's do it again, going back." Every one of the group got back into the fun of it again. Once the laughter and shouts of child-like cheer quieted down, someone asked: "What is the purpose or the benefit of it?"

The purpose of participating in child-like activities, either as a group of adults or as an adult with a group of children is that it makes one feel young again. It is well known among people who practice Laughter Yoga that children laugh 300 to 400 times per day. Studies show that adults on the average laugh no more than 17 times a day. The benefits of laughter are summed up in the old saying:'Laughter is the best medicine.' Children's joy and laughter are contagious. Hence when playing with children as an adult or when doing child-like activities we will laugh more than usual. Laughter releases endorphins, our body's natural stress relief hormones.

The benefits of the Lipo-roll are many-fold. Primarily it simply is fun to do and it will make you laugh, whether you do it by yourself or with a small group of friends. The extra benefit is that rolling on the ground surface increases circulation and breaks up cellulite, those unsightly fatty deposits under the skin on the hips and buttocks. There are more significant therapeutic benefits to rolling. Rolling improves coordination. It promotes and retains balance. Also, it can benefit neuromuscular control.

https://www.ncbi.nlm.nih.gov/pmc/articles/PMC2953329/

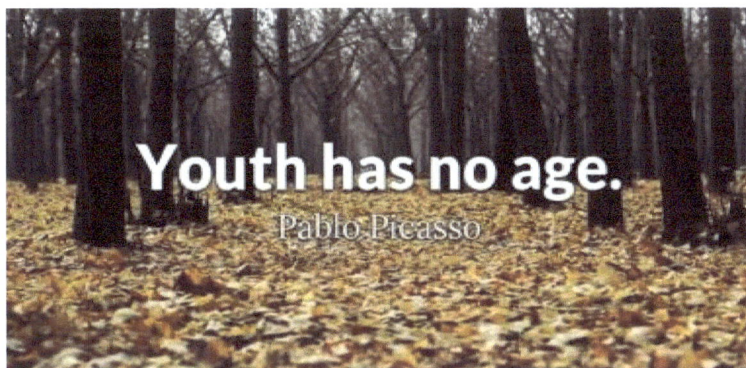

Youth has no age.
Pablo Picasso

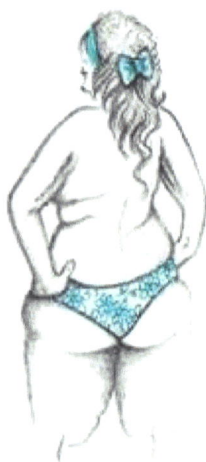

"My worth is not measured by the size of my waist."

Working on Areas of Concern

Do you have any unwanted body fat
on your inner thighs or under the buttocks?
Do you have varicose veins that bother you?
Do you have saggy underarms or crepey skin?
Do you have flabby flanks or a bouncing belly?

Concerns about one's body image are for real for both men and women. When I started with Quantum Body Sculpting, I was under the impression that the emphasis would automatically and mainly be on the body shape of women. I was somewhat surprised to read that statistics quoted in the Men's Health Section of the Guardian Magazine indicate there is more widespread anxiety about the way their bodies look among men than among women. Studies that were done at the Centre of Appearance Research at the University of the West of England support that there is increasing concern about body image among men. Terms like 'beer belly' and 'man's boobs' or 'moobs' are derogatory about of the male physique. Women tend to want to be shapely and slim, and men want to be big and lean. The media and celebrities influence us all by unhelpfully reinforcing unrealistic ideals of physical perfection. I'll be the last one to say that wanting to look good is a bad thing. My emphasis is that there are natural means to help ourselves to look good and feel good about our appearance. We can look good, not primarily to impress, or to become a glamorized image to be whistled at or adored. Our goal is to look good, so we can feel good and be empowered to do good.

I have selected to work on some particular areas of common concern about body image. We offer energetic correction techniques that involve energy work, such as focus, intention, and a positive attitude. The methods we provide, by themselves, may not be sufficient to come to grips with possible underlying causes.

The procedures work best when done in combination with an active lifestyle and healthy diet. It also helps not to take yourself too seriously. A sense of humor lightens things up. Enjoy! Have some fun. I guarantee there will not be any non-beneficial side effects.

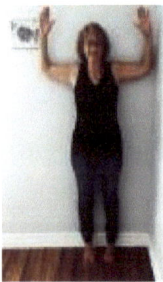

The pictures in the section on 'Areas of Concern' are pictures of myself at my current age, 79, taken by my husband with his cell phone. The intent is not to show photographic skill, but to encourage you that with a healthy diet, reasonable exercise and Quantum Body Sculpting the human body is happy and able to maintain an anatomically correct and proportionately pleasing shape. If I can do it, so can you.

104

Flabby underarms

Possible causes for flabby underarms are sudden and massive weight loss, being overweight or having suffered muscle loss. The purpose of the following technique is to

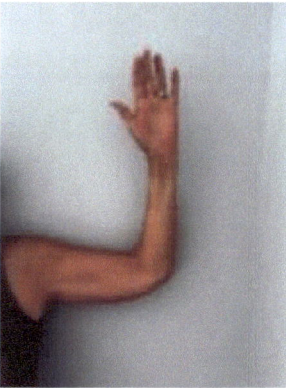

regain muscle strength in the upper arms. The benefit is that you will feel better when wearing sleeveless clothing again. You will likely become able to carry heavier objects again and to more easily take items off and put them back on to the top shelves in your kitchen cupboards or workshop storage areas.

Set your intention each time you do the technique: "It is my intention to firm up the muscle tissue in my upper arms." Repeat some of following positive affirmations or make up your own.

"I have strong and healthy muscle tissue in my upper arms."

"I look good in a sleeveless top and a short sleeve shirt."

"I love the way my body looks."

"I am healthy and well."

"It is fun to improve my appearance."

105

Quantum Body Sculpting Corrective Procedures

Before starting the technique take a few moments to find your quiet space using meditative breathing. Connect to the Life Force Energy as explained under the 'movements and exercises' section above. You can do this technique sitting or standing.
Cross your arms and place the palm of your hand on the underarm of the other arm.
Hold the positions and run energy for 5 minutes.
Do the same for your other arm.

You can do this technique while watching TV. You can do it while riding the subway or a bus to work and at any time of day when your hands are free and you can find a few minutes to focus on it.

Crepey skin

Possible causes for crepey skin are the loss of collagen and elastin in the underlayers of the skin. The crepey look of your skin may be a sign of chronic dehydration. Some people blame the natural aging process for crepey skin and learn to live with it or dress to cover it up.

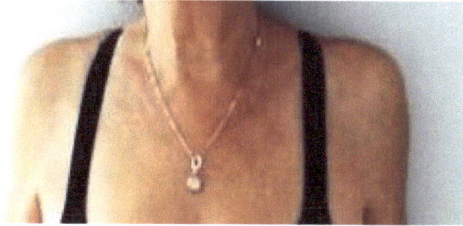

The purpose of the technique is to boost the growth of both elastin and collagen in the skin. The benefit is that you look and feel better in your skin. You will feel free to wear shorts, tank tops, and short-sleeve shirts again in warm weather.

Set your intentions: "It is my intention to rebuild collagen and elastin in my skin. It is my intention to have smooth skin on all parts of my body." "It is my intention to drink enough water regularly."

Internally say positive affirmations to yourself while doing the technique:

"I have beautiful skin on my arms and my legs."

"I love the way my skin feels and looks."

107

"My skin sparkles."
"My skin is healthy, and it looks youthful."

Quantum Body Sculpting Corrective Procedures

You can do the technique while standing, sitting or lying down. Begin meditative breathing and connect to the Life Force Energy.

Place the palms of your hands on the affected areas. Hold the position for 5 minutes or more while running energy. There are numberless opportunities to practice this technique during an ordinary day of your life. Here are some suggestions.

You can do it on your hands while attending a lecture or while listening to a concert or even while waiting for your turn in a dentist or doctor's office. Place your hands in your lap and do the technique on your thighs or place one hand on the other while focusing on youthful looking hands. Practice the technique on several areas of concern while watching a movie for example.

Spider and varicose veins

Excess blood which may bulge the surface leg veins ranks first among the possible causes of varicose veins. Hormonal changes may weaken the valves in our leg veins, then blood tends to leak backward. When the blood pools it can cause the veins to dilate and bulge. Standing still in one place for long periods at a time may be a contributing factor. Gaining weight may also create their appearance. Aging and pregnancy tend to get a lot of blame. They may contribute, but are not the sole causes.

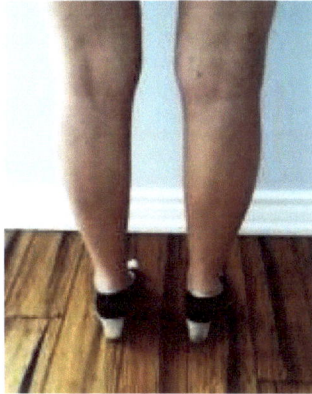

The purpose of the QBSc technique is both preventive and corrective. Doing the procedure on spider veins can prevent the development of varicose veins. You will

109

strengthen the valves in the surface veins. Also, it may thin the blood or prevent clotting and the bursting of the veins. The technique will lessen the likelihood of complications and side effects such as swelling and bleeding.

The benefit definitely has cosmetic value. If you were embarrassed to show your legs because of varicose veins, you'll now be pleased to wear shorts again. You'll be free from concerns about having to wear supportive hoses. But more than that, the technique will improve the quality of your life by preventing, reducing or eliminating aching, throbbing, heaviness, itching, or cramps.

Set your intentions. "It is my intention to repair the valves in the surface veins on my legs. It is my intention to eliminate all spider veins from my legs. It is my intention for my blood to flow freely through the veins on my legs."

You can internally say some positive affirmations while doing the technique:

"I have beautiful legs."

"My veins are healthy and well."

"It is fun to be able to wear shorts and mini skirts again."

Quantum Body Sculpting Corrective Procedures

You may do the technique while sitting or lying down. Begin meditative breathing and connect to the Life Force Energy. Place the palms of your hands on the affected areas. Hold the position for 5 minutes or more while running energy.

It is a good idea to practice this technique every evening before going to sleep. If you cannot reach your calves with

110

your hands, imagine you have longer arms and place your imaginary hands on your calves. You can also put your hands so that your palms are open and facing towards the affected areas.

Knees, calves and ankles

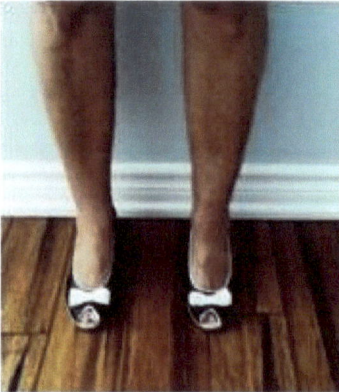

Fluid buildup, excess fatty deposits, or inflammation are probable causes for swollen knees, calves and ankles. There may also be possible causes at a deeper physical and psychological level. It is likely for healing to happen there as well.

The purpose of the correction is to remove inflammation and reduce fatty deposits from your legs, knees and ankles. The benefit of doing the QBSc techniques on your knees, calves and ankles is a reduction of swelling and inflammation and having shapelier and toned legs.

Set your intentions: "It is my intention to regain and to retain proportionally pleasing and anatomically correct body shape. It is my intention to have legs that are well toned."

The following positive affirmations may be repeated internally while doing the techniques.

"My legs are well toned."

"I like my legs; they are doing an excellent job getting me from place to place."

"My lymphatic system is working optimally."

"I am committed to maintaining an active lifestyle."

"My knees and ankles can support my exercise program. It is fun to be able to exercise."
"I am committed to eating a healthy diet."

Quantum Body Sculpting Corrective Procedures

It is best to do the techniques while sitting in a comfortable position in a recliner or a zero gravity chair. Begin with meditative breathing and connect to the Life Force Energy. Place the palms of your hands on the affected areas. Focus your attention on your lymphatic system. In your imagination visualize your legs to have proportionately pleasing shapes. Hold the position for 5 minutes or more while running energy.

Inner thighs and under the buttock bulges

Possible causes for inner thigh and under the buttocks bulges include fat pockets build up, unproportionate weight gain, lack of exercise, or too much icing on the cake.

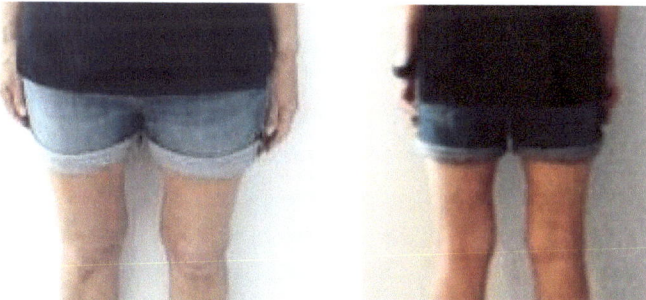

The purpose of the technique is to break up the unwanted fatty deposits on the thighs and buttocks. The benefit is an improvement in your body image and better fit in more snugly fitting jeans.

Set your intentions: "It is my intention to dissolve fatty deposits on my buttocks and thighs."

"It is my intention for my body to have a proportionately pleasing shape."

Some positive affirmations are:

"I love my shape."

"My clothes fit me properly. "

"I enjoy wearing snug fitting clothing with ease and comfort."

Quantum Body Sculpting Corrective Procedures

You can do the technique while sitting, lying down or in some cases while standing. Begin meditative breathing and connect to the Life Force Energy. Place the palms of your hands on the affected areas. In your imagination visualize your thighs and buttocks to have proportionately pleasing shapes. Hold the position for 5 minutes or more while running energy.

You can do this procedure while watching your favorite TV program. You can do it every night before falling asleep. You can do it while taking a shower. You can do it for 2 minutes every morning when getting dressed. You can do it in your imagination almost at any time of the day.

114

Love handles or flabby flanks

The most common causes of love handles and flabby flanks are an unhealthy diet and lack of exercise. Stress, as well as lack of sleep may also be contributing factors. For women, deep emotional issues may cause love handles in spite of eating healthy and exercising regularly. The purpose of the technique is to re-shape your midsection and to remove any unwanted fat build up. The

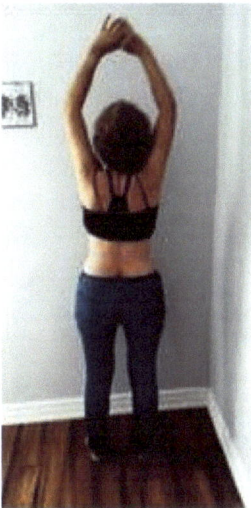

benefit is that you will no longer have to hold your breath while buckling your jeans. You will look better. You will feel better about yourself.

Set your intentions: "It is my intention to have a trim and well-toned midsection." The following positive affirmations may be repeated while doing the technique.

"I have a well-toned midsection."
"I enjoy a good night's sleep every night."
"I love the way my body looks."
"I love it when my clothes fit properly."

Quantum Body Sculpting Corrective Procedures

You can do the technique while sitting, lying down or in some cases while standing. Begin meditative breathing and connect to the Life Force Energy. Place the palms of your hands on the affected areas. In your imagination visualize a trim and firm waistline. Hold the position for 5 minutes or more while running energy. Ask your heart for advice to improve your lifestyle.

There are endless opportunities to practice the technique during an ordinary day in your life. You can do it in the theater or at a concert. Try it for a few minutes in the morning before getting out of bed. Do it at night before going to sleep and don't worry about falling asleep while doing so. The effect will linger, and you may even have happy dreams about a shapely you.

Sagging breasts and moobs

Weight issues likely are the dominant causes of sagging breasts. Double breasts may be the result of poor fitting bras. Both problems often become aggravated by stress or lack of sleep. There may also be emotional issues that impact the size and shape of your breasts.
Women readily tend to blame gravity.
Men breasts or moobs often are just fatty tissue. If you are otherwise in good physical shape and breast tissue develops it may be an indication of hormonal unbalance and your testosterone levels may be off. In some cases, man breast tissue may be indicative of liver problems, kidney failure or an overactive thyroid.

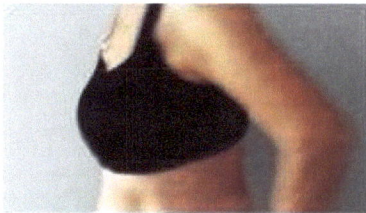

The purpose of the technique is to firm the breast tissues and muscles and to bring them to anatomically correct and proportionately pleasing body size. The benefit is that you will feel good about your body shape.
Set your intentions: For women: "It is my intention to firm and tone the tissue and muscles of my breasts." For men: "It is my intention to have a healthy and muscular chest."
Here are some positive affirmations to use.
For women:
"I love the shape and size of my breasts."

"I have perfectly proportioned breasts."
"I love the way I look."
For men:
"I have a strong masculine chest."
"My chest muscles are well toned."
"I am in great shape, and I like the shape I'm in."

Quantum Body Sculpting Corrective Procedures

The technique may be done while sitting or while standing. Begin meditative breathing and connect to the Life Force Energy. Imagine yourself looking your very best. Place your open hands under your armpits. Hold the position and run energy for about 5 minutes.

You can do this procedure any time you are at a concert, in the theater, or watching television. You can do it while waiting for the subway or the bus.

Bouncing belly or beer belly

Among the possible causes for a protruding belly digestive issues and fluid retention rank high. For women it often is difficult to bring stomach muscles back into shape after a pregnancy.

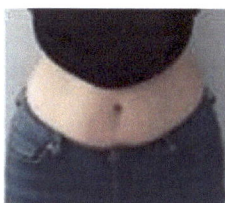 Secondary causes include fat deposits and emotional issues.

The purpose of the corrective technique is to strengthen abdominal muscles. The benefit is a flatter tummy for women and a more masculine

physique for men. You will feel better. Any possible digestive issues likely will ease significantly.

Set your intentions: "It is my intention to have strong abdominal muscles." "It is my intention to have a flat tummy." You may use the following positive affirmations.

For men: "I love my masculine physique."
For women: "I love having a flat tummy." "I am happy with the way my body looks."

Quantum Body Sculpting Corrective Procedures

You may do the next technique while sitting, lying down or in some cases while standing. Begin meditative breathing and connect to the Life Force Energy. Place the palms of

119

your hands on the affected areas. In your imagination visualize a trim and firm belly. Ask your heart for advice on how to improve your lifestyle. Hold the position for 5 minutes or more while running energy.

You can do this procedure any time you are at rest. You can do it one-handedly while you are scrolling up and down your computer screen. You can take a minute to set the procedure, place imaginary hands on your belly and set the intention. Set it and forget and go on with your other activities. Double tasking is no problem.

Timeline therapy

Timeline therapy may be done at the end of each corrective technique on areas of concern. While doing meditative breathing with your focus on the area of

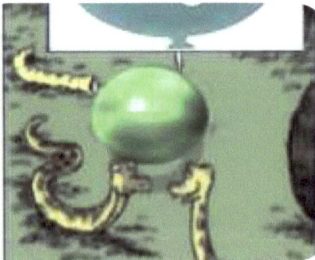

Why don't you change back into the skin you had when we first met?

concern in your body, do the following method. Go back in your memory to a time in your life when your body shape was the best shape that you can recall. Recall how you felt about yourself. Bring back the full experience of your life at that time. Visualize how you looked and sense how you felt. Did anyone compliment you on the way you looked? What did they say? How did you respond? What did you tell about yourself? How did you feel about yourself at that time? What were some of your favorite activities to do at that time?

Internally answer the questions. Answer in full sentences and include the emotions you felt at that time of your life to your answers.

How would you like to look and feel that way again five years from now? How about looking and feeling that way two years from now? Next year? Next month? Next week? How about right now?

Visualize looking your very best in your current wardrobe. In your imagination go shopping for a new and better fitting outfit. Visualize the new you at your current job, meeting your current friends and family. Describe the way you look. How do you feel? What do people tell you? How do you answer them? Are there some activities that you cannot do now, which you'll be able to do when you look youthful again? Imagine yourself doing those activities again. Enjoy!

Imagine it. Sense it. See it. Feel it, and Make it Real.

Take care of your body. It's the only place you have to live.

Jim Rohn

Working on Body Systems

Up to now, we have practiced meditations, movements, elongations, and exercises. We made corrections to particular areas of concern. All of those techniques are effective to sculpt our bodies. For the sculpting to be genuinely useful and for the results to last, more needs to be done. We need to work from the inside out as well as from the outside in.

Our body systems all work together to make us who and what we are, how we function and how we look. In the next section of the QBSc program, we will work with energy procedures on several of the human body systems to boost and support the work we have done up to now.

The combined use of intentions, meditations, positive affirmations and running energy allows us to influence the way our body systems work. One does not need to have a lot of background in energy work to be able to do the techniques. The directions are clear and easy to follow. The positive outcomes will usually manifest themselves immediately. It simply is the way our bodies work. Our body, our mind, and our heart listen to us, listen to each other and can work in perfect coordination, collaboration, cooperation, coherence and integration of our overall wellbeing.

If any of the procedures feel strange or if it is difficult for you to go on an imaginary journey through your body, no worries. Just try it or imagine doing it. Alternatively, go on to the next procedure. Make sure to take a break between doing any of the following procedures. Perhaps do one per day until the process becomes familiar to you. Trust your intuition to guide you concerning the way you can use the program for your highest good. Give it a try.

Experiment.
Wonder.
Enjoy!

Toning the skin

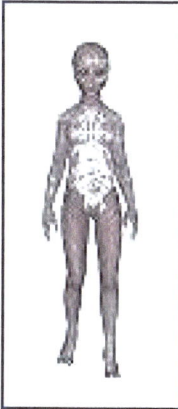

The skin is the largest of all our body systems. However, it does not usually receive equal recognition as a body system compared to the respiratory, circulatory or other body systems. It is not hard to believe that good looking skin is part of our body image. The skin on our face and the skin on our hands play a significant role in creating the first impression we present to our family, our friends, or colleagues and co-workers, and to everyone we meet.

The purpose of the following procedure is to smoothen and firm up your skin. The benefits are that your skin will become well-toned and you will have a more pleasing appearance.

Set your intention: "It is my intention to use my body's innate intelligence together with the intelligence of the Life Force Energy to tone, smoothen and firm up my skin now." You can use the following affirmations.

"I have healthy and beautiful skin."

"I love the color of my skin."

"My skin is well toned."

"My skin provides me with a pleasing appearance."

125

The procedure

You can do the procedure while sitting or lying down in a
relaxed position with your hands resting, slightly cupped and
comfortable, palms upward and tilted somewhat towards each
other. Begin with meditative breathing and connect to the Life
Force Energy. Drop into your heart space. Breathe and in your
imagination have a look at your skin. I do not mean that you
stand in front of a mirror to look at your skin. Look at your skin
with your eyes closed. Does your skin look and feel the same
all over your body? Do all parts of your skin look the same?
Do they feel the same? Focus on the temperature. Focus on
the texture. Has it always looked and felt this way? How would
you want it to look? How is it supposed to look? You can focus
on the areas of your skin that concern you most. You may see
or feel some irregularities. If you do, in your imagination
carefully prod an irregularity and find out if it can change. Ask
if it will change. Direct your energy and the love of your heart
to your skin. Imagine it and see it as being healthy, beautiful
and well-toned. Hold this thought and continue breathing
slowly for 5 to 20 minutes. You may feel a slight prickling all
over your skin. You may feel warmth in the palms of your
hands. You may feel nothing at all. That's OK. Enjoy doing
something good for yourself. If your thoughts tend to wander,
that's normal. Bring them back to the feeling of your skin, and
recall your intention. Continue breathing slowly.
You may do this procedure as often as you like. You can do it
before going to sleep. You can do it during a coffee break. You
can do it at home. You can do it when riding on public

126

transportation. You can do it with your eyes open or with your eyes closed.

If something comes up that interrupts you and needs your attention, don't worry. Tell yourself: "The energy can continue working while I do something else." In other words, you "set it and forget it."

Correcting and strengthening the skeleton

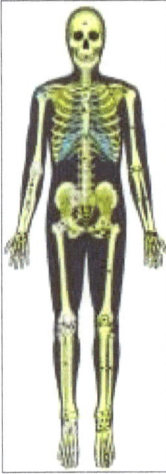

Our skeleton provides the framework for the shape of our bodies. For any sculpting on our body to be sustainable, we have to make sure that the framework is in good shape.

The primary purpose of the procedure is to maintain or regain bone density. The secondary intention is to adjust some bones and joints, hips, knees, the occipital ridge and shoulders in case they are slightly out of alignment. The benefits are that you will have stronger bones and a better posture.

Set your intentions: "It is my intention to strengthen my bones so they can give me a good posture." "It is my intention to maintain or regain bone density as appropriate for my body's size and weight." You can use the following intention for the second part of the procedure. "It is my intention to use my body's innate intelligence together with the intelligence of the Life Force Energy and my heart's energy to adjust my hips, occipital ridge, knees, and shoulders to return to their natural healthy and anatomically correct state."

Positive Affirmations.

"I have strong and healthy bones."

"I have an excellent posture."

The skeleton procedure, part one

You can do the procedure while standing, sitting or lying down in a relaxed position with your hands resting, slightly cupped, palms upward and tilted somewhat towards each other. Begin meditative breathing and connect to the Life Force Energy. Drop into your heart space. Breathe while in your imagination you have a look inside your body at your entire skeleton. Begin with a bird's eye view. Look at your complete skeleton. Look at the shape of your bones. Do they have a form similar to the pictures of skeletons you have seen in anatomy books? Try to get a sense of their texture. Look inside your bones. Do all your bones look the same? If you see anything that seems a bit unusual, wonder if it is supposed to look like that? Try prod the 'out of order' part and wonder how it can change for the better. Send your love and send your energy to that area. Continue breathing slowly for 5 to 10 minutes, then send gratitude to your skeleton for supporting you. When you sense you have taken enough time with your bones, bring the session to an end, and go on with your day's activities.

You can do this procedure as often as you want to. It is best to do it at a time and in a place where you will not be interrupted. Pay attention to how your body feels. Pay attention to the way you move and walk when the session is complete. Have any changes taken place? Take note of and compare any changes when you do the process again.

The skeleton procedure. Part two

The following procedure is for misaligned hips or to check if they are misaligned. Also, it is appropriate if someone has ever told you that one of your legs is longer than the other. Maybe it is, or maybe it isn't. Do it standing barefoot on a regular carpet or a yoga mat. Stand tall, with your feet approximately shoulder-width apart, knees relaxed and slightly bent. Start meditative breathing and connect to the Life Force Energy. Place your hands on your hips, palms slightly touching your body and fingertips pointing down at a comfortable angle. Set your intention to adjust your hips, occipital ridge, knees, and shoulders to return to their natural healthy and anatomically correct state for the highest possible good now. Breathe slowly and wonder what will happen. Do not apply pressure. You will likely begin to sway a bit. Allow it to happen. It is your body correcting your posture. When you stop swaying, the procedure is complete. It should not take more than 5 to 10 minutes.

You can do this procedure at any time, anywhere, whenever you sense your posture needs adjusting. Do it after a fall, after participating in any strenuous physical activity of any kind, or as a routine health check.

You can do the same procedure, rewording your intention and affirmations as appropriate, to adjust your occipital ridge. Do this if your mirror shows you frequently hold your head at an angle. When working on the occipital ridge, place your thumbs in the two hollow places, or dents at the bottom of the back of your head. Adjustment of the occipital ridge usually only takes a minute or two.

Shaping up the muscles

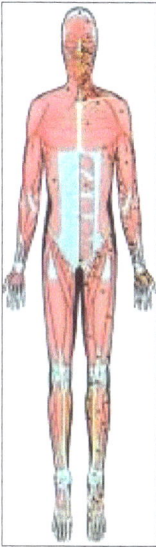

The primary function of the muscular system is the ability to create movement. Muscle tissue is the only tissue in the body that can contract and thus move the other parts of the body. Related to the function of movement is the maintenance of posture and body position. We have three types of muscle tissue. For body sculpting, we will focus on the skeletal muscle tissue.

The purpose of the procedure is to strengthen the skeletal muscles and to make them more flexible to carry out movement for all bones, to support the body and to maintain correct body posture. The benefit is that you will be able to have good posture and walk gracefully.

Set your intention: "It is my intention to use my body's innate intelligence together with the intelligence of the Life Force Energy to **anatomically** correct my posture from the bottom of my feet to the top of my head." "It is my intention to release all tension, relax my body and revitalize my muscles to the highest performance level for my body now."

Positive Affirmations.
"My muscles are healthy and strong."

131

"I exercise, stay active and eat well to keep my muscles healthy and strong."
"My muscles can provide me with good posture."

The procedure

It is preferable to do the procedure while lying down in a relaxed position with your hands resting, slightly cupped and relaxed, palms upward and tilted somewhat towards each other. Begin meditative breathing and connect to the Life Force Energy. Drop into your heart space. Breathe and in your imagination have a look inside your body at all your skeletal muscles. Start with a bird's eye view. Look at your entire muscular system. Look at the large muscles in your legs, the muscles in your arms, the muscles on your back. Do they look like the pictures of muscles you have seen in anatomy books? Try to get a sense of their texture. Look at the smaller muscles as in your hands and feet, in your neck, around your ribcage. Do all your muscles look the same? If you feel any tensions in a particular tissue, breathe into that area. Ask your muscles to let go of any stress. When you sense you've been able to release as much tension as possible at this time, the procedure is complete for that area. If there are other tense areas, you may go on and breathe into them. Alternatively, you can do it at a next session.

You can do this procedure at any time you feel your body is tense or stiff. Do it before or after a workout at the gym. Do it before and after engaging in strenuous physical labor. Do it as routine fitness practice.

Easing up your digestion

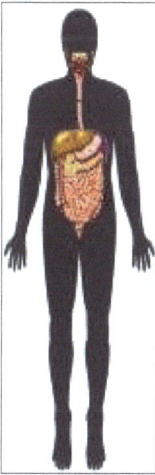

The function of the digestive system is to break down and absorb the food we eat to provide us with energy and to sustain our body. It consists of the gastrointestinal tract and several minor organs. For body sculpting, we are dealing with the process of digestion in general terms. We also focus on a few of the accessory organs, the liver, and the kidneys to assist in natural detoxification. Eating healthy and natural foods is a prerequisite to promote easing the digestive system.

The purpose of the procedure is to boost the proper functioning of the digestive system and some of the accessory organs.

The benefit is that you will have stronger abs and a flatter tummy. If you have swollen ankles, this process may well bring them back to normal.

Set your intention: "It is my intention to use my body's innate intelligence together with the intelligence of the Life Force Energy to absorb the nutrients from the food I eat and nourish my body and release all toxins."

Positive Affirmations.
"I commit myself to eat healthy and wholesome foods."
"My body can digest the food I eat."

"I trust my eating habits to supply my body with all the nutrients I need."
"All the organs of my digestive system work well."
"My digestive system helps me to have a proportionately pleasing body shape."

The procedure

Do the procedure while lying down in a relaxed position. Place your hands, palms down on your abdomen. Your hands need to be relaxed. Make your touch ever so light. Begin meditative breathing and connect to the Life Force Energy. Drop into your heart space. Breathe and in your imagination have a look inside your body at all the parts of your digestive system. Imagine some food entering your mouth, imagine chewing and swallowing. Follow the process of eating, digesting and eliminating as if it is happening in a movie on fast forward taking 5 minutes from start to end.

If you see any areas of tension, breathe into them until you sense the pressures are released as much as possible. Imagine yourself having a perfect body shape. Do this for 5 to 10 minutes.

You can do this procedure in connection with the bouncing belly correction technique.

Appreciate or re-activate your glands

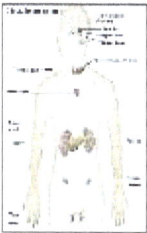

The glands control many bodily functions including drive, emotions, growth, energy production and the repair of damaged tissues.

Proper functioning glands tend to reduce stress and normalize energy levels. Working on the thyroid may normalize the release of hormones that govern weight issues. The pancreas regulates secretion of insulin into the bloodstream to regulate blood sugar levels. Hormones from the parathyroid glands help control calcium and phosphorous levels.

The purpose of this procedure is to boost your glandular system so that it can work at optimal capacity to support the body sculpting exercises you are doing. Benefits are that your stress level will go down. Your bones will regain proper density in proportion to your body size. It will become easier to maintain a good build and body shape. Set your intentions: "It is my intention to use my body's innate intelligence together with the intelligence of the Life Force Energy to optimize my glandular system's functionality, to release negative energies, balance my hormones and maximize positive energies throughout the glandular system."

Positive Affirmations.

135

"All my glands work at optimum capacity."
"I have a healthy hormonal system that works well to maintain an anatomically correct and proportionately pleasing body shape."

The procedure

Use heart energy to boost your glandular system. Sit in a relaxed position.
Drop into your heart space. Breathe and in your imagination have a look around your body, at your glandular system. Run energy, in other words, send the love of your heart and your appreciation to your glands to help reduce stress and to help your body maintain a good build and shape.
Do this for 5 minutes on a regular basis, once or twice a week.

Engaging the love of the heart

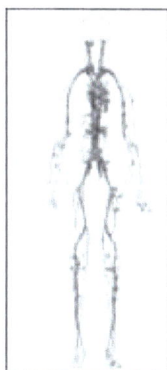

I refer to the heart in each of the mediations and in all of the comments about breathing while doing the exercises, movements, elongations, as well as in the corrective work on areas of particular concern. In all of the Quantum Body Sculpting work we engage the love of our hearts to send care, appreciation and, where appropriate, healing to our bodies. The heart is the control center of our body and connects us with our life experiences. Recent research on the priority of the heart shows that the heart is more than just a pump. It is. In the following section on the circulatory system, I focus on both the heart's intuitive intelligence that provides us with information, insight, and guidance in our lives and a system that relays information to the brain, as well as the heart's function as the center of the circulatory system. When our heart and brain are in coherence, we experience more ease in our lives, allowing us to project a positive body image.

A heart centering meditation

I invite you to do the heart centering meditation at any time you feel in need of being more positive about yourself.

137

The book *The HeartMath Solution* by Doc Childre and Howard Martin describes in detail how this meditation can be used to relieve stress as well as painful emotions. I've chosen to include it here because it has value in boosting your self-esteem and hence supports a positive body image.

For the duration of the meditation arrange not to be disturbed. Take a comfortable position, close your eyes, and relax.

Start breathing in and out more and more slowly. As you do this imagine or visualize that your breath is going directly through your heart. Do this for a few moments.

Think of someone whom it's easy for you to love and cherish, such as a friend or a child. Start to focus on the love you have for them. Think of times you looked at them. Remember the sound of their voice and your voice speaking to them. Think of times when you held them or were held by them. Think of touching them tenderly. Think of being touched by them. Keep thinking of all of the exchanges of love and appreciation with this person. Do this for five minutes or as long as fifteen minutes. If outside thoughts drift into your mind, gently let them go and draw your attention back to breathing through your heart. Then go back to your love for the person of your choice.

If external emotions intrude, or you feel blocked in feeling the love, picture your heart softening. Tell yourself it's not essential that everything needs to go perfectly every time. It's okay just to be learning the exercise. Breathe through your heart and see, feel, or imagine your heart becoming soft. Ask yourself: "What would it be like to be soft and yielding and totally relaxed?" It's okay if it doesn't all happen perfectly the first time, just try. You are doing something important for yourself. It's okay.

Now, go outside yourself and see or imagine yourself sitting there, in your relaxed position, doing this exercise. Take the love that you have felt for the other person and send it to yourself. Do this for up to five minutes. Imagine yourself with a pleasing well-sculpted body image.

Now send the love to others. First, send it to other people you find it easy to love. If you feel ready, you can try sending the love to others, even to people it's difficult for you to like. If you can't quite handle that, say to yourself, "I want to be able to feel this love and send it to this person. Meanwhile, I am willing that they will receive it from God or my higher self or the universe." Just be willing and open to having them receive love.

When you are ready, feel, picture, or imagine yourself completely wrapped up in a blanket of love for some time. Write down your experiences, intuitions, thoughts, or feelings of inner peace. Tell yourself that you are going to remember to act upon these feelings in your daily life.

cf: http://www.spiritofmaat.com/archive/nov1/hmath.htm

Cleaning the arteries

The purpose of the procedure is to clean the arteries to optimize circulation of the blood. The benefit is that you will be and feel healthier. You will be able to be more fully engaged in life with more energy and vibrancy. As a result, you will look better.

Set your intention: "It is my intention to have clean arteries and veins." "It is my intention to optimize my circulation." "It is my intention to use my body's innate intelligence together with the intelligence of the Life Force Energy to cleanse my blood, create new healthy cells, to release that which is no longer serving me. Instead, I will experience love, compassion, and longevity."

The following favorable affirmations may be used. You can also make up your own.

"My heart, arteries and veins are healthy and well."

"My healthy heart allows me to be active and well."

"I have good circulation and can now stand upright and walk with ease."

The procedure

You can do the procedure while sitting, or lying down. Begin meditative breathing and connect to the Life Force Energy. Place your right hand on your heart, and hold your left-hand palm up, ready to receive the Life Force Energy. In your imagination take a journey through your circulatory system. Follow the flow of your blood from your heart to all the extremities of your body. If you see any obstructions, narrower spots, unusual things or irregular flow, ask yourself: "Is this how it's supposed to look?" "Can it change?" "Should it change?" If the answers that come to you indicate a change is appropriate, take your imaginary finger and gently prod the unusual stuff you observe. Wonder and watch what happens. Send all your love to that area. Breathe into that area. Trust the process. Continue the procedure for five to ten minutes or more while running energy.

When complete, have a drink of water and resume normal breathing.

Following your heart's advice

The purpose of the procedure is to get in tune with the intuitive intelligence of your heart. The benefit is that you will increase your intuitive perceptions and learn to trust your intuition.
Set your intention: "It is my intention to trust my body's innate intelligence together with the intelligence of the Life Force Energy and follow my heart's guidance for my highest good." "It is my intention to have heart and brain coherence."
Some positive affirmations.
"I trust my heart's intelligence and guidance."
"I follow my heart's guidance about following the QBSc program so I can have the best body shape possible for me."
"I trust my intuition."
"It is safe for me to trust my heart and to trust my intuition."

The procedure

It is best to do this procedure at a time and in a place where you will not be disturbed.

Sit in a relaxed position, close your eyes and breathe a little more slowly than usual. Bring your focus to your heart. You can place one hand on your heart if that helps. Do this for 30 seconds. Now imagine your breath is going in and

142

out through your heart. Let go of all interfering thoughts and emotions, bringing yourself to neutral. You will likely feel less stressful and your heart rate will become more coherent, smoother. Think of some pleasant and positive events in your past and recall the emotions you felt. Relive those emotions, sense them and bring them into your heart space. Activate and sustain genuine feelings of appreciation and care. Continue breathing slowly with your focus on these emotions for two minutes. Ask your heart what is the most effective, the most beneficial way to deal with the current challenging situation. Wait for your heart to give you an answer. The answer may come immediately, but be patient, it may come later that day or the next day. Commit yourself to follow your heart's guidance.

You can do this procedure at any time and as frequently as you wish. Repeat it often until you can do it automatically and instantaneously. Then use it whenever life confronts you with a challenging and stressful situation.

"Like the sun, the inner Self is always shining, but because of negative clouds, we do not experience it. It is not necessary to program oneself with the truth; it is only necessary to remove that which is false. The removal of the clouds from the sky to illuminate the negative allows one to experience the energy fields of that which is positive. It is only the removal of the negative that is necessary-the willingness to let go of the habits of negative thinking. The removal of the obstacles to the experiencing of this will result in an increasing sense of aliveness and a joy of one's own existence."

~David R. Hawkins, MD, Ph.D

Appendix A
Applied Kinesiology - Muscle Testing

A brief explanation and an informal method to learn to do muscle testing. A complete description of the technique is beyond the scope of this book.

Muscle Testing is a component of Applied Kinesiology with its roots in traditional Chinese medicine. It is biofeedback, providing you with answers that aren't immediately available to the conscious mind. It includes information about energy blockages, the functioning of the organs, any nutritional deficiencies, any food sensitivities or allergies.

Muscle testing can also be used to do a check on limiting belief systems. It can be used to find out if a conscious belief agrees with the sub-conscious views that you are holding in your body ever since your childhood, or those from later in life.

 In case responses are inconclusive your energy may be blocked. You can do a polarity test and then correct the meridian flow. Sometimes all you need to do is have a drink of water, making sure you are not dehydrated. Muscle testing will not provide accurate responses to particular statements about the future, for example. You'll get a response, but if you say, "This answer is reliable," the response will be weak. Remember muscle testing is not a competition but a method to test for muscle strength.

How to do the procedure step by step:

1. Prepare for a muscle testing session with a few moments of quiet to become grounded.
2. Decide which method to use. If working with a friend, it is easiest to use the arm-test. If working by yourself use the O-ring or Thumb test.
3. Test for relative strength. How tight do you have to hold your fingers so as not to be able to pull out your thumb, or how hard do you have to push down for your friend not to be able to hold up her arm.
4. Test strength by using the following questions
• Please say: My name is (use your own name). Wait a few seconds and test. The response will be strong.
• Now say: My name is (use any imaginary name). Use a generic name of a person of the opposite sex. The response will be weak.
• Next test for Yes, Yes, Yes, and then for: No, No, No.
• Think of someone, something or someplace you like. When you are in the feeling of it, test.
• Think of someone, something or someplace you dislike. When you are in the feeling of it, test.
• Take note of your answers.

Practice with a friend. Practice by yourself.
First test questions for which you already know the answer. Then test for issues to which you do not know the answer. Practice with various objects such as:

• Smell a flower, then an odious substance.
• View a picture of country scenery, then an accident scene.
• Hold a favorite vegetable, then a sweet cookie.
• Next do a blind test. Take four food items, some healthy and some not so healthy and wrap them in identical packages. Ask a friend to 'scramble' the package positions. Touch the bags one at a time and test: 'The food in this package is healthy for me to eat.' Were the answers what you expected?

 Use your imagination and test for other things and ideas.

You may test your attitudes and beliefs about Quantum Body Sculpting.
• Test: 'The Quantum Body Sculpting program will work for me.'
• Test: 'I have limiting beliefs that will hinder my success in maintaining a youthful appearance.'
• Test: 'I hold negative emotions that interfere with an anatomically correct and proportionately pleasing body shape.'

How to apply the practice in your life.

You can use muscle testing in your daily life. The possibilities are endless. When grocery shopping you can test if a particular item is good for your health, or if it is genetically modified. When shopping for other things, you can test to find out if it is a good idea to make the purchase. Even when you are writing a resume to apply for a new job, test the wording you use. Is a particular phrase effective? If not, rewrite the sentence and check again.

147

"I was exhilarated by the new realization that I could change the character of my life by changing my beliefs. I was instantly energized because I realized that there was a science-based path that would take me from my job as a perennial "victim" to my new position as "co-creator" of my destiny. (Prologue, xv)"

~ Bruce H. Lipton, PhD
Author of 'The Biology of Blief'

Appendix B

Belief Busting Kinesthetics is a derivative of the modality Psych-K used in the Quantum-Facelift level 2 online course. I have added it here because it can assist in removing limiting beliefs that may hinder you in maintaining an appropriate body shape.

Practice, Enhancement, Reinforcement

Belief Busting Kinesthetics is a derivative of Psych-K, a branch of Applied Kinesiology. It is meant to bring balance and agreement between the conscious and subconscious mind; between the brain and the heart. It can free you from negative self-talk patterns that limit your potential. It can break habits of self-sabotage. Since it is our beliefs that control our lives, let's make our beliefs about aging positive. The good news is that you can change your limiting beliefs about your appearance.

Remember the subconscious mind does not understand negatives. Always use first person singular, present tense, positive statements. Example: 'I have an excellent body shape.' Never test comments like: 'I am not fat anymore.' In that case the subconscious picks up on fat and more and will accommodate you with more fat. So, don't go there, unless that's what you want. ☺

How to prepare for a Belief Busting session

1. Prepare for a belief busting session with a few moments of quiet to become grounded.
2. Muscle test for: 'The QBSc program will work to improve the way I look.'
3. Muscle test for: 'I am happy about the way I look.'
4. Muscle test for: 'It is possible for the skin on my face to regain (or to maintain) a youthful appearance.'
5. Write your own belief statements about your appearance, the way you want it to be, and muscle test for them.
6. Take note of your answers.
7. If you test strong for any of the positive belief statements, congratulate yourself.
8. Balance to obtain agreement to the statements that test weak. Always first ask and test: 'Is it safe and appropriate to balance for that now?'

How to balance step by step:

1. Pretzel Up: Sit up straight on a dining room chair. Cross one ankle over the other. Cross the opposite wrist over the other. Interlace your fingers and bring them under and up so that your pinky fingers rest on your breastbone. Close your eyes. Place your tongue against your palate behind your front teeth. Repeat the statement for which you are balancing, internally, again and again, until you feel a shift. Unpretzle.
2. Keep your eyes closed, place your hands in prayer position and your tongue on the bottom of your mouth. Take a few slow breaths. Place your hands with your palms down on your thighs, open your

eyes and look at the floor 4 feet in front of you. Take a few slow breaths.

Muscle test the statement again. You will likely test strong, indicating agreement between your conscious and subconscious mind.

3. Congratulate yourself. Yeah!

4. Balance each of the statements about aging for which you tested weak.

5. It is advised to verify the statements now and then. Since the subconscious is predominant over the conscious mind, it may take over again. You may have to balance more than once, or even several times over the next few months until you continuously test strong for your more positive belief statements about aging.

How to apply the practice in your life.

You can test for and balance other limiting beliefs.
Test and balance your attitudes about yourself.
For example:
'I love myself.'
'I deserve to be or to have (something).'
'It is easy for me to.' etc.
Test and balance about your relationships, about your attitude towards money, about success in your career, about the nutritional value of your food choices.

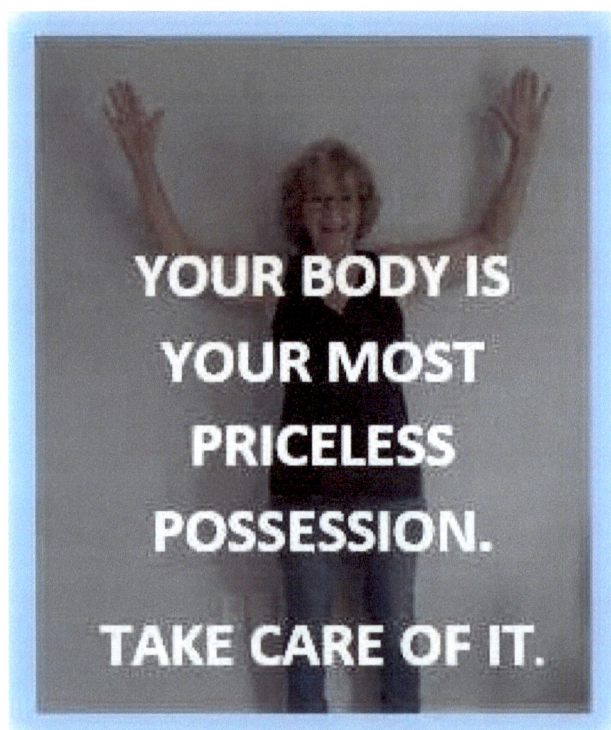

YOUR BODY IS
YOUR MOST
PRICELESS
POSSESSION.

TAKE CARE OF IT.

Conclusion

There are different ways to make use of the information in the book.

You may just read it, find it interesting material and put the book aside. If that is you, I am quite sure that in your imagination you have played with some of the movements, or elongations. You may even have tried an exercise or two. I expect at some time parts of it will resurface and you may wonder if it is worth your while to come back to the ideas and try to use them. In any case I appreciate the time you took to read it.

Some people may have experienced that some particular parts resonated with them and worked with those exercises, meditations or procedures that relate to their specific situation. If that is you, I'd love to hear from you about the level of success you have achieved.

Others may have read about what I refer to as 'running energy' for the first time in their life. If doing the procedures, movements, etc. felt useful to you, if you experienced any level of success, I congratulate you. I invite you to explore further to see what else can happen.

Perhaps you have become intrigued with the possibilities the alternative approach to taking care of your wellbeing has to offer, but you can not see a way clear to do it all on your own. If that is the case, I invite you to find a way to come to a workshop or a retreat so that you can learn and practice with others.

You may be an experienced energy worker and have used the same or similar techniques and methods for years. I trust you will enjoy my approach to using energy work as a method to maintain an anatomically correct and proportionately pleasing body shape.

Be Well!

Acknowledgements

I am genuinely grateful to have grown up in a family where alternative healing was the norm and where Dowsing was a part of life. Today I practice many healing modalities including Quantum Touch, Reiki, Psych-K, The Emotion Codes, Reconnective Healing, and Dowsing to mention a few. I am grateful to the Instructors of the ever so many workshops I have taken and how they have increased my skills and added to my understanding and awe of the miraculous power we have within ourselves to be healthy and well.

The methods used in the Quantum Body Sculpting work are a combination of ancient and modern healing techniques. Of all the healing modalities I have learned and practiced, there is none that has influenced me as much as what I have learned from the Institute of HeartMath. Several of the movements and exercises are similar to those used in Core Transformation. I thank Alain and Jody Herriott for introducing me to those techniques years ago.

Thanks to all my friends in Laredo, Texas for participating in the first run of the Quantum Body Sculpting workshop. Thanks to my healing friends Diane Michaud, John Compton and Kathryn Kimmins. Your participation and input have been immeasurably valuable. Thanks to Lee-Ann and Miriam Orta for perfecting all the movements and positions for the photographs. Many thanks to Nancy & Roberto Sandoval of Sandoval El Bello Arte photography for the excellent pictures you find in the book. I simply love the artwork contributed by my artist friend Nanci Stevens of Puerto Viejo, Costa Rica. You have an unbelievable eye for beauty. Last but not least, I much appreciate my husband Everett's editorial skills, his support and patience with me for all the time it kept me at my desk.

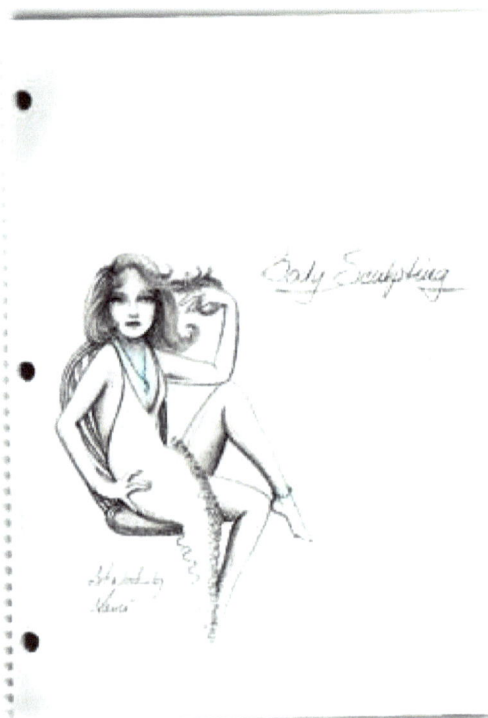

ArtWork by Nanci

My artist friend Nanci Stevens has an eye for beauty.
It is my wish that the QBSc program can help everyone to
sculpt their outer appearance to match their inner beauty.

Medical Disclaimer

I have taken utmost care to explain the methods and procedures to the best of my abilities. I offer no guarantees. I can only assure you that I do my best to share what I have to offer. The rest is up to you. Although each of the methods I use is highly effective in promoting one's body to restore itself to maximum health and shape, it may not be sufficient intervention for some health-related issues or non-beneficial diet and lifestyle practices. The program is not intended to be a substitute or replacement for qualified medical advice, diagnosis, or treatment. Quantum Body Sculpting works best when done in combination with a healthy diet and an active lifestyle. The sessions may also accelerate healing of body shape related as well as some other medical issues. If you are on medication, I recommend you work closely with your physician to monitor your need for drugs, with the intent to reduce your dependency on them. The information in this book is not intended to be a substitute or replacement for qualified medical advise, diagnosis or treatment. I am not engaged in rendering professional or medical advice.

No Limits

Most people experience some immediate improvement in their body shape as a result of the techniques I present. However, the sculpting process is highly personal. Results vary a great deal from person to person, even while using the same procedures and methods for similar issues or conditions. Some people experience immediate and stunning results. From my personal experience, it took commitment and continued practice to manifest fitness and wellbeing. I do not know the limits of what we can accomplish with a strong and confident intention. Give it your best, have fun, and allow your body to respond.

Please take responsibility for the shape you are in!

About the Author

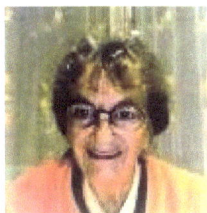

Trudy Baker has international experience as a Quantum Healing Instructor. After retirement, she returned to work full-time turning what was a hobby into a full-time career. She writes, presents workshops, and sponsors retreats. 'Healing from the Heart' and 'Come Breathe With Us,' are self-help books to encourage you to take responsibility for your own health and wellness, using techniques from many alternative healing modalities. 'Energetic Pampering: Quantum Face-Lift,' applies the same techniques to enhance your complexion. "Quantum Body Sculpting" is a comprehensive program of movements, procedures, and meditations for a complete body make-over to captivate the joy of ageless living. Beautiful from the inside out.

Books by Trudy Baker

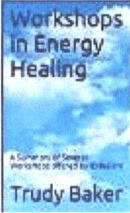

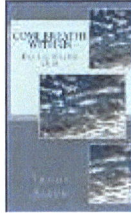

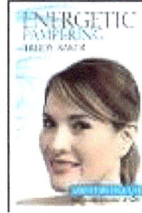

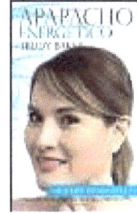

Online Course

https://courses.quantumfacelift.com/practice/qfl-users-guide/

Websites

www.quantumfacelift.com

www.ShifaHouse.com

www.IEHealers.com

Be Well!

Be Beautiful!

Be You!

162